Practical Handbook of Veterinary Homeopathy

Healing Our Companion Animals from the Inside Out

Wendy Thacher Jensen, DVM

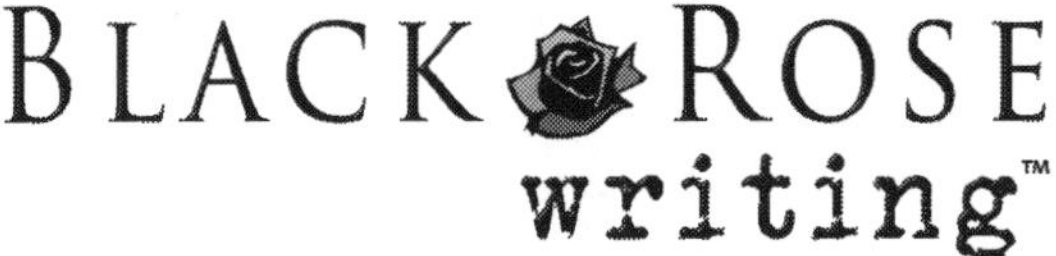

The final approval for this literary material is granted by the author.

First printing

This book is not intended for use by animal caretakers in treating their own companions. The author and publisher cannot be held responsible for unsupervised treatment. This book is designed to educate the animal caretaker. An informed consumer greatly increases the likelihood of a positive outcome, when working with your veterinary homeopath.

ISBN: 978-1-61296-612-0

PUBLISHED BY BLACK ROSE WRITING

www.blackrosewriting.com

Printed in the United States of America

Suggested retail price $16.95

Practical Handbook of Veterinary Homeopathy is printed in Garamond Premier Pro

Special thanks to Margaret Jensen for cover photography and interior artwork

Acknowledgements

Many thanks to my teacher, Dr. Richard Pitcairn, who guided me onto the one true path, and to Nicola Henriques, who kept me there. Thanks also to Dr. Christina Chambreau, who first opened my eyes to the wonders of homeopathy. To Doris Eder, a big smile, because she gave me the courage to keep writing. My deepest appreciation to the special animal caretakers whose words grace these pages and whose animals were my teachers. Lastly, I dedicate this book to Edward, who reminds me of all the other animals whose lives could be made better with homeopathy.

Practical Handbook of Veterinary Homeopathy

Table of Contents

Introduction

This book is written for our animals, who trust us with their safekeeping. To keep them healthy, we turn to modern medicine, but it is ill-equipped to address chronic disease in our animals and ourselves. We have become dependent on pharmaceuticals to address every ailment, one at a time. There is a different way. What if we as animal lovers could change our focus from individual symptoms to an awareness of the whole animal and their innate ability to heal? Then we would be well on our way to making our beloved companions' lives a lot better.

How do our animals get sick? What actually drives all these reactions, what invites in the bad bacteria, what allows the viruses to replicate, what turns the cells cancerous, what switches on the hurtful genes that produce disease? There is a glue that holds it all together, or a pilot, so to speak, a director of each individual animal and person. This thing suffuses every body, every organ, every cell, every strand of genetic material. It directs the flow of life and healing. This is the life force, our vital energy, our *wesen*, as it is called in the old books. If we get sick, our *wesen* has gotten sick first. If we spike a fever today, our *wesen* had already been disturbed long before. If we inflame our liver, it only happens well after our vital force first felt the impact of disease. Cancer comes only after this energetic imbalance thoroughly permeates our entire physical body. You can see the lump, but you can't see that the whole patient is sick.

Remember the story of four blind men touching a different part of an elephant, and each one relating a completely different experience? The tail, the trunk, the leg, the ear, and taken in isolation, each part suggested a completely different animal. Once I stepped back and realized that the teaching I had received in veterinary school was to medicine just as the tail is to the elephant, the shock was profound. I wanted to open my eyes and see the whole thing. But in order to do this, I had to re-evaluate everything I had learned and translate it into a new language. It took me awhile, but the work was well worth the effort. I learned that if I fought disease at the level of the vital force, I was fighting a war that could actually be won. But if I kept working at the outskirts, treating each symptom as if it was the sole cause of my patient's distress, I was doomed to failure, or at best an uneasy and temporary truce. I was the cartoon character mopping the floor next to a mysterious black box spouting tidal waves. If I mopped fast enough, I had moments of dry floor before I had to pick up the mop, wring it out, and start over. Now, I have found a better way. Share my journey, read this book, and find out how to open up the black box and turn off the spigot.

So what treats disease at the level of the vital force? What strikes illness at its source? What medicine can treat the *wesen*, at the energetic level, where both disease and healing begin? To answer, first I'll continue my story. After leaving the veterinary practice that sheltered me in my early years, I became a housecall vet. Happy to be on my own, but still wielding the same tools: antibiotics, prednisone, and hormones. My patients kept coming back to me sicker than before, perhaps healed from their original maladies, but now with more serious diseases I could not heal, such as hyperthyroidism, renal failure, and cancer. What was wrong?

First I decided that it must be my clients. I had not educated them enough. They didn't understand how to care for their animals at home. So I worked hard to ensure that all my treatment recommendations were being followed. I left no stone unturned. If there was a handout, I sent it home. If there wasn't any written information, I wrote it myself. I talked to everybody about proper diet, training, healthy environment, and good breeding practices, until I was talked out and had no more to say. Nothing changed. My patients came back sick anyway. Then I decided it must be my practice's treatment policies. I was trying to handle diseases that were beyond my skills as a general medicine practitioner. So I began referring clients to specialists, hoping for healthier patients, but no, the results were not encouraging. My patients came back to me with bags full of ointments and pills, detailed handouts and diagnostics describing their illnesses, along with their still-unchecked diseases. Managed, yes, but inexorably progressing until the end. Who was left to blame? Me? It couldn't be my training, because I had graduated from one of the best schools in the country. I kept thinking and wondering.

Then one day I was invited to a lecture on homeopathic veterinary medicine. I was mildly curious, but not prepared for the experience to follow. What was this about a vital force? About how disease began at the energetic level and only then moved to the functional level, then on to pathology? As each point was made, all the pieces began to fall together. This made sense! A way to practice that cut right to the heart of the matter. Such joy! If I could learn to treat the imbalance in this thing called the vital force, then I could treat the disease rapidly, gently, and permanently. I could finally achieve my dream of true healing. I went on to take more in-depth classes and I have never looked back. I found what was missing in all my years of training and practice: a coherent, cohesive philosophy of medicine.

There may be the seeds of doubt in you as well, which is why you picked up this book. Do you notice unique things about animals or people that set them apart from each other? Do you wonder why our friends and family members only add to their pile of prescriptions over the years, never really getting free? Do you love your veterinarian but wonder why the same problem in your animal keeps coming back again and again? Have you met the person who avoids doctor visits? Why would they do such a thing? Because they are not happy with the results. Homeopathy can do far more for your animals than symptomatic treatment, and you are the key to the best possible outcome. That is because your observations and knowledge of your animal are the key to your homeopath's success.

• • •

As a high school student, I walked dogs at a local veterinary hospital. Since I also cleaned the kennels, everything was easier if my charges eliminated outside. I took care to encourage this. During my time spent in this practice, I began to realize that each patient was unique. The way they greeted me, their manner of walking on the leash, how they investigated their surroundings, how they chose the proper spot for elimination, how their body moved during the act, what they did afterward. Some were happy no matter how sick, cheerfully licking my hands and sniffing each flower. Some were grumpy, preferring to eat before they were walked, or relaxing only if I stroked them carefully in that perfect spot before we headed out the door. Other differences were more physical. Some were troubled with straining during their bowel movements, and among those some strained before anything was produced, others after everything was done. For a kennel girl, the former required patience whereas the latter could simply be carried back to the kennel with impunity. The poop itself varied amazingly, even among patients on the same hospital food. Different color, degree of odor, consistency, size, amount, and so on. At the time I was just interested in getting the poop onto the grass so it wasn't left in my clean kennel, not realizing that noticing these differences would be so crucial to my work as a homeopath, years later.

I also had doubts during veterinary school, which I rapidly squelched because after all what could I know, as a mere student? I had spent way too much money on tuition to question my professors at this late date. One patient who left me unaccountably saddened was the heavily sedated German Shepherd weakly straining out a bit more enema fluid onto the floor of his kennel. He was awaiting a colonoscopy. I kept returning to clean him up, wishing there was more I could do to ease his misery. I wondered how important it could be, this plan to visualize the insides of his intestines. Could we really help him just by looking at the lining of his gut? And the microscopic analysis of any lesions found there--this is still, in essence, vision. So the cells are changed from epithelial to cancerous. How really does that inform us of his disease? Of how the dog himself was sick? And what does it tell us of how to make him well? All these diagnostics do not tell us how the entire patient is sick. I wondered about this early on, not knowing that I was coming close to another important truth. Years later I would learn that we cannot see disease itself, only the pathology that is disease's endpoint. Cutting out all the cancer does not remove the disease from the patient. Disease begins well before the first cancerous cell grows, and disease is still present after all the cancerous cells are removed.

If this gets your attention, consider this book an introduction, an eye-opener. Read it if you are ready to choose a new path for the health of your animals. Learn how to be the eyes and ears of your veterinary homeopath. Not every patient who comes to homeopathy is healed, as many come so terribly damaged from years of medications. Sometimes the best your homeopath can do is to ease a patient gently into a quiet peace before the end. But many can be saved. With our newfound vision, our new understanding, together we can listen to each patient and allow them to direct our actions. I no longer fight my patients' symptoms in order to make them better (while only driving the disease deeper). Now I speak the language of the vital force and use the symptoms as a guide. It's a partnership that only gets better with time and experience, and I want to share it with you. I want you to know what it looks like when medicine is practiced in a logical, coherent manner, with overriding principles that guide each step. The vital force reacts to disease in definite, discernible and predictable ways. If all modern veterinarians and physicians and animal caretakers understood the philosophy behind homeopathic medicine, we would have powerful tools for healing. Now I can help my patients heal at a much deeper level, treating the vital force directly, experiencing the partnership that I only imagined I was playing into during my Cornell experience. Now I am living it for real. But I need the help of my clients, clients like you, to do my best.

Throughout this book I will be quoting from the most important text containing the principles of homeopathic philosophy, the *Organon of Medicine*, by Dr. Samuel Hahnemann, as well as other sources. This book was written in the late 18th century by a physician who had left his medical practice after becoming disenchanted with its violence and often less-than-salutary results. While translating a text on the successful treatment of malaria with cinchona, or quinine, Dr. Hahnemann found himself disagreeing with the author's explanation of the mechanism of cure. So he took cinchona himself and found that he, as a healthy person, experienced the same symptoms as patients with malaria! In proposing that the symptoms caused by medicines in well people also cure those same symptoms in sick people, Hahnemann had re-discovered the principle of "like cures like." He was not the first scientist to discover this principle, but he was responsible for developing it into a medical art. This proving, or determining the action of drugs in the healthy body, was the first step towards a system of medicine based on pure observation, rather than conjecture. Now, thanks to Hahnemann and his followers, we have books, called materia medicas, full of provings of hundreds of substances, and we also have the understanding to apply this knowledge towards the cure of our companions. We no longer have to treat symptomatically. "Usually not knowing what else to do, the old school has always tried to combat and wherever possible suppress through medicines *only one* of the many symptoms that diseases present--a *short-sighted method* called symptomatic therapy....A single symptom is no more the whole disease than a single foot a whole man."[1]

What does this mean? It means that the whole patient is treated, not just the tumor or the thyroid gland or the kidneys. After all, the body is connected to the thyroid, and medication used to alter the thyroid's function has effects on the entire body. We live as a whole body, intricately connected throughout its parts, from the external-most skin to the internal-most nerve cells. Homeopathic philosophy enables us to treat disease and, whenever possible, achieve cure of the entire patient, from skin to neurons.

Enjoy the following cases from my practice, as a taste of homeopathy in action. (Throughout this book, the names of the patients have been changed to protect the client's privacy.) See how the whole animal is affected, not just a symptom. Notice how infrequently the medicine is given, and also how the entire patient improves, not just the most worrisome symptoms. Then go on to study this book. As an educated consumer, you will greatly increase the success of your homeopath. You are the key to improving your animal's health.

Use this book according to your own needs. If you are here to learn everything you can about homeopathy, you will probably enjoy every chapter and page. You will get a solid grounding in homeopathic philosophy while gaining a deeper understanding of the work that goes on after the patient intake is complete. If you are just getting introduced and want only a taste, you may prefer to spend time with the first two chapters, then skip ahead to read the illustrative cases at the end of most chapters. These cases highlight the wonderful possibilities of homeopathic treatment. Most of the cases are dogs and cats, since they make up the majority of my practice. Regardless, the philosophy and methods apply to all species, including humans. (For information on natural equine care, Dr. Joyce Harman is a good resource at http://harmanyequine.com/.)

A Horse with a Melanoma

Katrin, a 21 year-old grey Arabian mare, had a pool-ball-sized melanoma at the base of her jaw, diagnosed with a needle aspirate. Her guardian had tried the traditional anti-tumor treatments with another horse and had not been satisfied with the results, so she came to me and asked for homeopathy. Over a period of several months and a few doses of her remedy, the tumor slowly shrank, finally leaving her cancer-free and enjoying walks in the woods.

Old Cat with Hyperthyroidism

Yizzy, at 20 years old, was on multiple medications for hyperthyroidism, chronic renal failure, asthma, constipation, vomiting, and a poor appetite. She also had a lung tumor. With only two doses of her homeopathic remedy, over the next eight months, her caretaker was able to get Yizzy off many of her medications. She stopped vomiting, began eating better, and best of all, her lung tumor began shrinking, before she was lost to follow-up.

Cat with Inflamed Gums

George began life as a stray, and when he finally lucked into a good home, he was suffering from terribly sore gums, putrid breath, and a bad cold. Homeopathy not only cleared up his cold, but totally resolved the inflammation in his mouth. Before treatment, George had never meowed, and now he has found a voice!

Dog with Dysplasia

Stan was easy to walk, even as an excitable 10 month-old Golden Retriever. He would barely put any pressure on the leash, waddling with his tail tucked way down, even dragging his feet. His hips were severely dysplastic (deformed) and he was facing corrective orthopedic surgery. He also had a thick black ear discharge. After homeopathic treatment, his tail came up like a flag, and his ears cleared up. He became very strong, even powerful. Stan no longer needs hip surgery. This case shows that even though our animals can be born with a genetic disease, homeopathy can ease their symptoms and enable them to live a healthier life.

• • •

Introduction Reference

1. Hahnemann S. *Organon of Medicine, Sixth Edition.* Künzli J, Naudé A, Pendleton P, eds. Blaine, WA: Cooper Publishing;1982: 13.

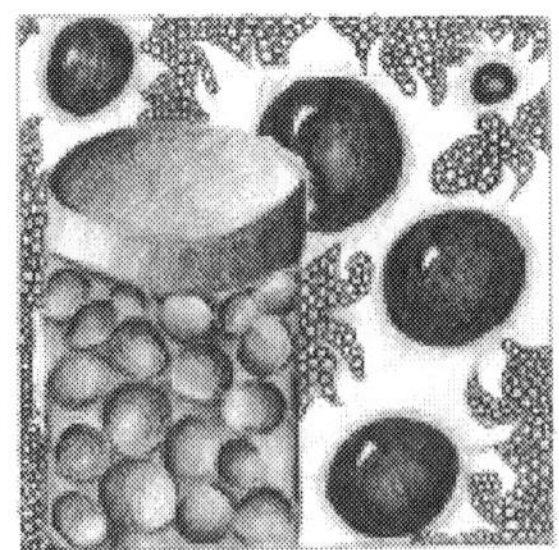

1 - Why Should I Study Homeopathy?

"The highest ideal of therapy is to restore health rapidly, gently, permanently; to remove and destroy the whole disease in the shortest, surest, least harmful way, according to clearly comprehensible principles."
—Hahnemann, A. 2, *Organon*

Why study? Why learn this new way of healing? Study because it takes time to change your inner focus from particular symptoms to the whole patient. In order to heal our animals, we need to do more than treat symptoms. Did you know that there is only one organizing force in the body responsible for healing? When the body swings into action to heal a wound, this power is the same that responds to a cold or an infection. There is only one. It works as a single unit, directing the immune system, the nervous impulses, the blood flow, and the cells of the body in order to get and keep the body well. Even the will and the thoughts are directed by this force. The bladder doesn't have a separate immune system from the skin or the ears or the brain. The immune cells do not originate in the stomach or the eyes.

Did you know that the body does not get sick in individual parts? When the bladder is inflamed, the whole body is sick. Even though symptoms may only express themselves in the bladder, this portion of the anatomy is not isolated from the rest of the body. The body works as a whole, and when one of its parts is expressing symptoms, the whole body is ill and disorganized.

Did you know that symptoms tell us the body is sick, but that symptoms are not the sickness itself? Symptoms only tell us the nature of this particular illness in this particular body. Think of the words of a familiar song:

Rock-a-bye baby, in the tree top
When the wind blows, the cradle will rock....

Are these words the song? Which words? Cradle? Bough? Tree top? Perhaps all the words are important, like—blows the when wind? Or is the order important? When the wind blows. Is that the song? No. The song is the words, in the proper order, with the proper spacing between the words, at the right pitch of the music, and sung with expression and emphasis on certain syllables. BA-by, not bab-BY, right? The symptoms are no more the disease than the words are the song.

What about smelly ears, with a thick brown waxy discharge, and an itch? Are the ears sick? In order for the ears to have these symptoms, the whole dog had to be sick first. His illness is the pitch and the melody and the phrasing, *along with* the words.

Did you know that if we stop a symptom, we are not curing the patient? It's not the same. Stopping the symptom only prevents the patient from expressing his disease. Anti-biotics, anti-inflammatories, anti-nausea drugs, these all are given to stop a single symptom. The disease as a whole, the imbalance, though still present, becomes indiscernible, until another symptom or set of symptoms is expressed. The illness song is still playing in the patient—we just can't hear the words anymore.

Symptoms are the words of a song, but they are not the song itself.

Did you know that symptoms in one part of the body are expressing the same illness as symptoms in another part of the body? A hypothyroid dog with a hotspot has one illness. The thyroid is not in charge. The hotspot is not in charge. The patient's healing force is sick, and it is a unit.

Did you know that a sick body needs only one medicine in order to heal? There is only one disease in a sick dog or cat, so they need only one medicine to get better. Once the healing force, or the vital force, is engaged, then all symptoms get better. Not just the ears or the thyroid or the bladder, but all the parts get better together. This is true healing.

Did you know that homeopathy improves the health of patients over the years instead of just healing the current illness? This medicinal system prevents future health problems, even such minor indispositions like bad breath, smelly skin, or furballs. And homeopathy has no side effects. The body responds as a unit to medicines. There is no true hierarchy of real effects and side effects. If a medicine is properly chosen to match the entire illness, all of these different "side" effects match what needs to be corrected in the patient. Healing proceeds naturally and completely, engaging the entire vital force of the patient.

"*The physician is...a preserver of health if he knows the things that disturb it, that cause and sustain illness, and if he knows how to remove them from healthy people.*"—Hahnemann, A. 4, *Organon*

So why study homeopathy? Study so that you can learn what it takes to engage the vital force of your companion animals. Study so that you can help your animals live healthier lives. Study because our animals need us. In nearly 30 years of veterinary medical practice, I have witnessed a growing tendency among veterinarians and physicians to rely on physiologically active doses of medications to treat our patients' ills. "Physiologically active" means that the medicine consists of concentrated substances that interact directly with the chemical processes in the body. For example, insulin lowers glucose levels, cortisone inhibits inflammatory mediators, and aspirin fights fever-producing prostaglandins (compounds produced in the body). Unfortunately, this near-sighted focus on individual symptoms assumes that disease consists of high blood glucose or itchy skin or a fever, and that the rest of the patient, apart from the problem, is well. This emphasis on one aspect of the diseased patient fosters the misconception that correction of that aspect is curative. Modern medicine says the entire problem is with the tiny insulin-producing cells of the pancreas. That liver disease means a sick liver, but the rest of the patient is well. Or in the case of an itch, once ruling out mites or other external causes of itching, the only "treatment" is cortisone to suppress the itch. A scratch-free dog is considered cured, until the next cortisone injection is required. Likewise, in human medicine, an adult patient with a fever is given aspirin as quickly as possible to bring the fever down.

Symptoms are only the visible manifestations of disease.

Our entire body consists of interconnecting chemical pathways with attendant checks and balances. If one blood value is altered, or one chemical pathway is blocked, or one symptom is artificially altered with drugs, repercussions are felt throughout the organism. As any master clockmaker knows, we simply cannot change one small spring in the clock without impacting the entire machine. As we lower the glucose, stop the itch, or drop the fever, the body changes in other ways, and the changes are not always beneficial.

These changes are often given the broad label of "side effects."

Side effects are unintended and usually undesirable reactions of the patient to a treatment regimen directed at a single symptom.

Side effects are a natural consequence of changing one part in a multi-part system. "Other than the possible side effects, what's the problem with this approach?" you might ask. Chronically elevated glucose levels have serious health consequences, such as cataracts, compromised kidney function, and a deranged appetite. Therefore, normalizing the glucose level seems a worthy goal, at first glance. A chronically itchy dog will suffer from inflamed abraded skin, infections, and broken sleep. Fever is also quite uncomfortable with its attendant aches and pains, even causing seizures in susceptible individuals. So why not address these issues?

• • •

There is a better way. We can stop the itch and have a healthy dog. We can remove inflammation without suppressing the immune system. I'm not recommending that we just let our animals suffer. This medicine, homeopathy, addresses the body's illness in all its complexity. This medicine reverses the disease process simultaneously along every altered pathway. Imagine a ball of yarn caught by a cat's claw. You extract the claw and retrieve your ball, finding a long loop pulled out of the center. You can stuff the loop back in, apparently fixing the problem, but that will leave many tightly-pulled strands buried inside. The yarn ball is no longer the same. Homeopathy can loosen those tight inner strands.

Another way to picture giving a medicine which addresses only one symptom is to imagine pulling the arm of a person relaxed on a sofa, until the limb is outstretched along the top of the cushion. You have pulled so hard that this person tilted a bit in your direction, head leaned to one side. After getting a complaint, you insist that you can get your friend back to his former comfortable position without his help. So you put his hand back in his lap, you push on his head to center his neck, and you press on his shoulder. Have you returned him to his original position? Likely not. Most likely there are muscles up and down his back that are still twisted, inaccessible to your hands. If he gave up on your help and moved himself, he would use multiple muscles and ligaments and tendons throughout his body to straighten himself. He would not need to look at every displaced muscle, or pay attention to every body part. This return to equilibrium would be natural and rapid, thoughtless even.

Imagine a medicine that could return the ill body to homeostasis, or a state of healthy equilibrium; a medicine that dives right into the distorted ball of yarn to ferret out every tight strand, returning every loose loop to its former tension. Conventional "fix the symptom" drugs can't find everything that's out of order and fix it without creating havoc. But our animal patients can do the work of healing themselves, if we use medicines that enable their innate abilities.

"A single symptom is no more the whole disease than a single foot a whole man."
—Hahnemann, A. 7, *Organon*

For 200 years, homeopathic physicians and veterinarians have been treating their patients based upon ALL their symptoms. This means that there are no side effects, because all of the effects caused by the medicine help with the healing process. One medicine covers all the symptoms, and all the effects of the medicine help with all the symptoms. The state of the organism in disease, including all the symptoms, is matched with a remedy that stimulates the entire organism to return to balance. How is this done? You are the key. You are the best person to learn to identify your animal's symptoms and evaluate their response to treatment. Studying this book and other books on homeopathy will enable you to work with a veterinary homeopath to deeply heal your animal family members. The following chapters will explore how homeopathic veterinarians discover the proper remedy for their patients. At each step, you will learn how to assist your veterinarian—how to give them the best information about your animal. Homeopathy recognizes that each patient is different, whether suffering from the same diagnostic label or not. One diabetic cat will need a different remedy than another diabetic cat, and each itchy dog or fevered cow will require a remedy based on their unique combination of symptoms, rather than their disease label.

My aim in writing this book is to educate you, the consumer, so that you can recognize the goal of true health and the means to attain that goal. How does a practitioner take a good case? What do they do with this information once it is received? What kinds of reactions will you see in your companion animal? If animal caretakers learn to recognize quality in homeopathic medicine, they will demand it of their veterinarians. (And physicians!) Health care practitioners, when faced with educated clients, will seek out training in homeopathy in greater numbers, and medicine itself will change its focus from the symptom of a disease to the patient as a unique whole.

What needs changing isn't the cell in the pancreas that produces insulin, rather it is the animal as a whole who has become sick. The animal who can no longer produce her own insulin, the patient who reacts to multiple common allergens, the feverish patient, all need medicine which restores balance to their complex inner workings. Our patients need medicine that addresses the entire imbalance at once, not piecemeal, and you are the perfect one to encourage this change. So study on, and enjoy the journey!

• • •

Here are a few more cases from my practice to enjoy. We will study cases in more detail in later chapters, but these are presented to celebrate the amazing changes possible with homeopathic treatment.

A Horse with Bladder Stones

Edgar, a 14 year-old Hanoverian, presented with recurrent bladder stones. Unhappily facing a second surgery, the clients sought out homeopathy. After a single dose of his remedy, his nearly golf ball-sized stone disappeared and he went back to upper level dressage work.

The Irritable Poodle

Zena, a 9 year-old Standard Poodle, was overly sensitive, reacting fearfully to her guardian's moods. She would guard toys from her fellow house mates, and bite at the least provocation. She didn't like getting wet, urinating on the sidewalk rather than stepping into a puddle. Her body was always tense, her limbs stiff and her head held high. She had a heart murmur. She didn't drink much and her mouth was always smelly. With homeopathy, she made a complete turn-around. She now runs into puddles for a drink, swims in the river, and plays hard with her dog friends. Her posture has relaxed, her heart murmur improved, and she no longer needs annual dental cleanings. Instead of growling and avoiding guests, she now solicits attention. She is a changed dog.

The Hyperthyroid Cat

When 13 year-old Tracey began feeling badly, her guardian had blood taken. Tracey was hyperthyroid. She was irritable, sleeping more and losing weight, and she had had a 3 mm pink growth on her head for the past four years. After her remedy, her thyroid hormone levels returned to nearly normal, she gained her weight back, her behavior improved, and the growth crumbled away into dust.

The Lame Dog

Princess the Labrador Retriever was brought in when she was nine years old and could no longer run to retrieve her favorite ball. She had pain in her back and a black discharge in her ears. After homeopathic treatment, she was back to chasing balls, and her ears improved as well.

Canine Chronic Diarrhea

Charlotte was a tiny Boston Terrier mix who suffered from diarrhea so severe it was affecting her growth. A change of diet only made things worse. Homeopathy resolved her diarrhea and now she is a finely-muscled, beautiful adult who can eat anything.

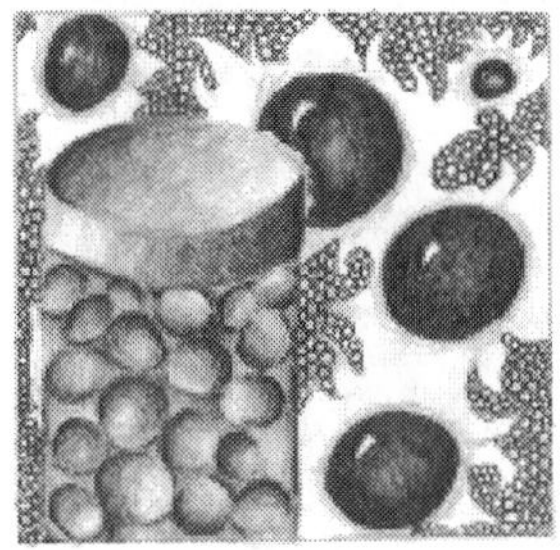

2 – What Does Homeopathy Heal?

What is Health?

Homeopathy is the body's catalyst for regaining health.

Homeopathy is a system of medicine that brings your companion into a state of health by supporting and directing the body's intrinsic efforts to heal itself. When one of my cases treated with homeopathy (after hours of study) turns a corner and things begin going well, clients commonly say, "I guess she just decided to get better!" Then I know that I have done good work, because homeopathic healing comes directly from the patient, and not from the medicines. Homeopathy treats at the energetic level. We are all beings moved, motivated, and directed by energy. That's where disease begins.

There is a children's story about a wager between the sun and the wind. Both wanted to remove the coat from an old man walking down the road. (The coat represents the man's disease.) The wind said, "I'll just blow his coat right off!" But the man only held tighter to his coat. So now it was the sun's turn. The sun simply beamed hotly down, and of course the man promptly took off his coat. Treating disease at the level of the vital force is like giving the man a good reason to take off his own coat. Homeopathy enlists the body's healing powers, and the result is a gentle, natural return to wholeness.

What is this state of wholeness anyway? Health. It's an easy state of being, free of pushes and pulls that limit our animals' full expression of themselves. It's a natural state that resists the disease-causing effects of bacteria and viruses, a sturdy base that keeps our animals going strong even under less-than-ideal circumstances. When healthy, our companions are free to just be. Most of us, and most of our animals, are not living in a state of health. This makes it very difficult to fully visualize what it means to be truly healthy. Most people think of health in terms of what ISN'T there rather than what IS there. For example, health to most of us means an absence of pain, or an absence of anxiety and sadness. Or the absence of physical difficulties such as arthritis or headaches, diabetes and weight problems.

True health goes well beyond the lack of symptoms.

The body free of disease is strong and vital, able and willing to exercise without pain. The digestive system works well, producing an appetite for healthy foods and creating the ideal weight naturally, without dieting. The senses function well, providing reliable information about our environment. The skin is clear and resistant to the effects of changes in environmental temperatures and humidity. The hair or fur grows well and is shiny and full. The respiratory tract is resistant to common viruses and bacteria, and does not react to allergens. The body is fertile and able to reproduce. The bones are strong even into old age, without medications. Sleep comes easily and renews the body and mind nightly. The healthy person is able to concentrate for long periods, free to relax and play, socialize, dream, and create beauty. Our emotions flow freely, allowing feelings which are expressed as needed during the course of a day, neither hurting nor hurtful.

Does this give you pause? It should. The more you study homeopathy, the more you come face-to-face with the realization that few among us are truly healthy. We need a better system of medicine. Homeopathy has the great potential to move many of us and our animals along the path towards true health.

What is Disease?

Disease is first and foremost an energetic distortion.

Now that we can visualize our goal, the next step is understanding that which needs to be cured. Since the symptoms are not the disease, we must look deeper. Disease is an imbalance or distortion of the energy of the body. When the body energy is treated directly, symptoms go away on their own. A fever disappears without Tylenol. Blood glucose normalizes without insulin.

The body is connected by bones, blood vessels, nerves, muscles, lymph vessels, subcutaneous tissue, and skin. The various bodily systems work in concert with each other, digestion slowing during physical exertion, pupils dilating when the mind is fearful, and blood pressure rising when the patient feels angry. The body and mind respond as a unit to any situation, whether it is a physical challenge or an emotional situation. Our animal's bodies and minds respond together to various kinds of weather, or social situations, or even the mental stimulation of learning a new skill. We and our animals are incapable of limiting our reactions to a certain body part.

Thus it is with disease. When the body is sick, even if the visible manifestations are limited to one area, the whole body is diseased. It is the energy of the vital force which needs help, not the body parts and their symptoms. Remember that German Shepherd from the Introduction to this book, awaiting his colonoscopy? He would still be sick, even if all his lumps were found and removed, every last little one. His illness was not limited to the areas of changed cells. He was sick throughout his entire body. That which is to be cured is energetic and involves the whole body, not just the abnormal cells.

Illness begins and is sustained at the energetic level.

We and our animals need help in the form of medicines that treat our energetic imbalance. In order to understand how homeopathic medicines cure disease, let's examine more closely the nature of disease and how it establishes itself.

• • •

Consider that you are coming down with an illness. You have no symptoms yet, but you know that something is coming on. You don't feel like yourself. This might be difficult to discern in your cat or dog—they might just pick a different sleeping spot or have a different expression on their face, like a canine patient of mine who furrows his brow. At this point, the sickness is at the energetic level. This is the root of all disease. No disease can exist in the body without having first permeated the energetic level. This first impingement of the vital force is invisible, impalpable, and immeasurable. (We will briefly discuss acute disease separately as it is a special case.) At this point, there are no symptoms. Nothing to see! Yet the body is sick. Then comes a change in sensation.

• • •

Energetic level → Sensation Changes

• • •

Now you definitely know something is wrong with your companion, because he is tired and droopy. Sensations are difficult to ascertain in our companion animals, but not impossible. You might pat your dog as you usually do when you come home, and suddenly he yelps and cringes away. Or that joyful walk that used to take a whole hour is cut short when he drags his feet, then sits down and refuses to move. You know something is wrong. Yesterday, everything seemed to be working within the normal swings of day-to-day variations. But today is different, and you can see it. Your companion is still sick at the energetic level, but now the illness has also risen to the level of sensation. There are still no measurable symptoms, but he is ill. This is the point at which you would consider bringing your cat or dog to your veterinarian and requesting diagnostics. The third level of disturbance is a change in function.

• • •

Energetic Level → Sensation Changes → Functional Changes

• • •

If you do not treat the disease when it reaches the energetic or sensation level, it progresses over time to what traditional medicine would now call illness. This is the functional level of disease. Functional disturbance follows and is concurrent with illness at the energetic and sensation levels. There are measurable changes, such as a fever, nasal discharge, diarrhea and vomiting, a skin rash, or joint inflammation. These are the vital force's attempts to regain balance. If you had laboratory blood work done, it would likely be abnormal. The illness that began at the energetic level has now affected the cells in your companion's blood, perhaps also her body temperature, and there are discharges. The bowel is no longer functioning normally, or the respiratory tract is congested and not exchanging oxygen well, or there is a cough. The changes caused by the illness are tangible and concrete. Finally, disease progresses to the level of pathology.

• • •

Energetic Level → Sensation Changes → Functional Changes → Pathology

• • •

If treatment has not been successful, the tissues now begin to change. The body has gone beyond simple inflammation and functional changes, and the cell makeup and organization have become abnormal. The organ architecture has changed. The skin or bladder wall has thickened, the heart muscle has dilated. A tumor might have grown. The disease may be incurable at this stage. This is the end result of untreated disease, which may have taken many years to develop. Homeopathy can still help at this stage, but the patient is much harder to treat and the end results may be less than satisfactory.

From energetic changes to changes in sensation to measurable changes in function to palpable and visible pathological manifestations, this is how disease progresses. Every case of chronic disease, without exception, develops along this pathway. The earlier the disease is treated, the easier it is to cure. Homeopathy treats at the energetic level, at the root of the disease.

"...*diseases obviously* are not *and* cannot be *mechanical or chemical changes in the material substance of the body...but are an exclusively dynamic, spirit-like untunement of life.*"—Hahnemann, A. 31, *Organon*

Acute Disease

This type of imbalance is caused by external forces such as trauma or poisoning or certain virulent infectious organisms. The progression from the energetic level to the sensation level to the functional level is rapid, usually within seconds (in the case of trauma) to hours (distemper). Homeopathy is very helpful for acute diseases, and the response is faster than to traditional drugs. Since this book mostly concerns the treatment of chronic disease, please refer to the reference section for some guides on the use of homeopathy for acute or first aid situations. During an emergency, don't wait to get your animal to the hospital. You may be confident you have the right remedy, but give it *while on the way* to the emergency clinic.

Chronic Disease

The body cannot heal chronic disease without help.

The O'Reilly edition of Hahnemann's *Organon* defines chronic diseases as, "...those which (each in its own way) dynamically mistune the living organism with small, often unnoticed beginnings."[1] These unnoticed beginnings are disease at the energetic and sensation levels. The body cannot heal chronic disease without help—it can only mitigate the damages by attempting to limit its sphere of influence in the body. For example, one patient may limit her most severe symptoms to the joints, thereby avoiding pathological changes in her liver or kidneys. Other patients might display their chronic disease mostly on the skin, with hotspots and ear infections. Chronic disease lasts for the lifetime of the animal, unless treatment addresses the underlying energetic imbalance that allows the disease to flourish. The body is unable to rid itself of an energetic imbalance without help.

How can disease last for years? Because at its beginnings, it is quite subtle and practically unnoticed by the vital force. As Hahnemann writes, "[Chronic diseases]...dynamically untune the living organism, each in its own way, and remove it from health gradually, in such a way that the automatic vital energy (vital force, vital principle) intended for the preservation of health can offer only imperfect, inappropriate, ineffective resistance to them, both at their start and as they continue, and can never extinguish them on its own, with its own power, so that it must impotently let them flourish while it becomes ever more untuned, until the organism is finally destroyed. We call these *chronic* diseases...."[2]

Chronic diseases are rampant today. We are all familiar with diseases that have labels, such as diabetes, kidney failure, and hyperthyroidism, for example. These, incurable with Western medicine, develop over time, with ever worsening pathology. This quote describes the pathology of diabetes: "The pancreas becomes firm and multinodular and often contains scattered areas of hemorrhage and necrosis. Later in the course of disease, a thin, fibrous band of tissue near the duodenum and stomach may be all that remains of the pancreas."[3] A cat suffering from kidney failure has small nodular kidneys, along with muscle wasting. Hyperthyroid cats have thyroid nodules and an enlarged heart.[4] Pathology is the ultimate result of chronic disease.

Disease starts at the energetic level and only over time becomes discernible to the patient, then visible to the practitioner, then finally obvious to the rest of the world. Inflammatory bowel disease, for example, illustrates disease that has reached the functional level. Many cases may also be pathological, with visible lesions in the intestines. But the patient with inflammatory bowel disease and its attendant appetite loss, diarrhea, and weight loss did not jump straight to functional and pathological illness. He was sick long before the first abnormal stool. This is the stage, before pathology, before a label, before a diagnosis, this is the stage at which treatment is most effective.

Illness begins at the energetic level, and here it is most easily treated.

The best way to help your animals is this: Learn to recognize the early signs of chronic disease. Then you can help your homeopathic veterinarian head off a lifetime of illness in your animal. Every sick patient has unique symptoms that begin well before functional disease. These early symptoms are not specific to a disease, such as diabetes, but are characteristic of each particular patient's illness. Once you know how to "see" disease before it creates pathology, half the battle is won. You will be able to significantly increase the health of your animals.

How is this possible? How can we recognize illness before the blood glucose goes up, or before the diarrhea begins? Simply this: We learn to recognize the symptoms of chronic disease that are present before pathology. These are not hard to see, though they are so prevalent now that we consider them basically normal. Even if just slightly uncomfortable and easily assuaged, however, these are the signs of an illness that will progress over time unless the disease is treated at the energetic level. Unfortunately, modern medicine has spent all its resources developing treatments which work directly against single symptoms, instead of treating the whole animal at the energetic level. Doggy odor? Give a bath. Constipation? Give drugs which stimulate the intestine. Ear infection? Apply an ointment. Furball vomiting? Laxative to the rescue. Homeopathy, on the other hand, goes deep into the constitution to root out the cause of disease, leaving the patient well and free of constraints to full healthy living. Digestion eases, appetite normalizes, aches disappear, and best of all, the medicine cabinet empties out.

• • •

To treat chronic disease in non-human animals, you and your veterinarian need to see its expression. Many conditions which we see every day are actually the beginning stages of chronic disease, and if you treat your animal at this stage, you have a better chance of improving their health over the coming years. But learning to recognize early signs of chronic disease is not easy, because we have all spent years accepting that certain discomforts are just a way of life and a normal part of aging, for ourselves and for our animals.

"...patients become so accustomed to prolonged suffering that they no longer pay much, if any, attention to the many smaller concomitant circumstances... considering them almost to be a part of their natural condition, almost health itself...."—Hahnemann, A. 95, *Organon*

The body tells us it is sick through headaches, irregular bowel habits, acid indigestion and heartburn, or premenstrual syndrome. These are signs of early chronic disease and an unhealthy vital force. Chronic recurrent sore throats or ear infections, colds that always settle into the chest, excessive dental cavities, acne, dry cracking skin, premature hair loss, cystitis (inflammation of the bladder), difficulty concentrating or sleeping, extreme shyness, craving for sweets, alcohol, or drugs, all these are early chronic disease.

Chronic disease does not go away on its own.

How many of these symptoms have you simply passed on as habits peculiar to certain people, or aging, or bad living situations, or bad hygiene? Certainly paying close attention to one's diet and personal health care will minimize many chronic disease symptoms, but eating well and brushing your teeth do not cure chronic disease. It is the same for our animals. No matter how well they are fed, exercised, and loved, chronic disease, once present, steadily chips away at our companions' health until finally it emerges as a full-blown medical condition with a label. What makes matters worse, is that chronic disease is inherited, and many of our patients are sick right from birth.

• • •

Here are some canine chronic disease symptoms masquerading as breed traits or poor training:

Chronic Disease Symptoms in Dogs—Mental/Emotional

fear of loud noises, thunder or wind
barking too much and for too long
irritability/aggressiveness at play
suspicious nature
timidity
licking things and people
laziness
eating dog stool
feet sensitive to being handled
being destructive
sensitive to heat or cold

Chronic Disease Symptoms in Dogs—Physical

"doggy" smell
attractive to fleas
dry, oily or lackluster coat
excessive shedding
easily tangled fur
waxy ears or chronic ear problems
mucus on stools
diarrhea with every change of diet
obesity

bad breath
poor, finicky, or excessive appetite
stiffness on rising
hip dysplasia (malformed hip joints)

• • •

Get to know these signs and symptoms, because recognizing them early on in your animals, especially the young, easier-to-treat ones, will help you and your homeopathic veterinarian provide the best care possible. Do not stop treatment until these signs are all gone, and begin treatment again when any of these signs re-appear. Don't wait until pathology develops. Here are chronic disease symptoms in cats:

• • •

Chronic Disease Symptoms in Cats—Mental/Emotional

excessive timidity
biting when stroked too long, irritability
playing too roughly
hysteria when restrained
laziness
clumsiness, inability to leap to high places
not covering stool in litter box or not using litter box

Chronic Disease Symptoms in Cats—Physical

freckles on the nose, eyelids, and ears
fragile claws
loss of whiskers
attractive to fleas
dry dull coat

excessive fur loss
waxy ears or frequent ear mites
poor grooming habits
excessive or finicky appetite
eating inappropriate things
sensitivity to milk
drinking water more than once a week (unless fed dry food—then cats drink daily or more often)
constipation or hard, dry stools
diarrhea with every change of diet
frequent vomiting, even if just fur
obesity
emaciation
bad breath
pale or red gums
loss of teeth

• • •

You might look at these lists and say, "Why bother?" After all, most of these symptoms are mild inconveniences that can be managed with a change of diet, or brushing the teeth, or a good trainer. But remember how chronic disease progresses? Even if these mild conditions respond to good care, the chronic disease remains uncured. Big diseases begin at the energetic level, progressing slowly over time into the level of sensation, as discussed above, and then to function and pathology. So the inconveniences in the lists above progress inevitably to outright illnesses. Every patient is different—some may sicken sooner and some may remain relatively well-balanced throughout their life, but every patient will get the maximum benefit from treatment in the early stages.

• • •

So what is our goal in treatment? To manage symptoms? No! Homeopathy goes way beyond this. Our goal is true health, which is the absence of any limitation on our companion's ability to experience life. We want our dogs to be strong into old age, hiking with us and swimming in the lake. We want our cats to spend their last years cuddling sweetly on our pillows, purring, not suffering through yet another fluid treatment for chronic kidney failure. Homeopathy is a great gift. By participating in this mode of health care, we gain a greater awareness of our beloved animal's state of health, and through this an increased respect for the wisdom of their bodies. Through study and utilization of this superb healing modality, you will develop a deeper connection to your companions. Then, perhaps for the first time, you will experience the beauty of healing without harm.

Allopathy, or Welcome to Side Effects

Medicine taken for a single symptom cannot cure the body.

Allopathy is a term used to describe modern medicine, or Western medicine. Allopathy literally means "different suffering," or, in other words, that the treatment produces symptoms which are different from the symptoms of the disease. So for example, aspirin, while it lowers fevers, also causes severe abdominal pain, intestinal bleeding, ringing in the ears, swelling of the tongue, trouble breathing, and more.[5] Check the list of side effects for any allopathic medication and you will find all the symptoms produced by that drug. The drug itself has been put into production because of its most common effect, but every drug has a large number of other often harmful effects on the body. As O'Reilly writes of allopathic medicines, "The symptoms produced by the medicine have no manifest...relation to the symptoms of the disease."[6]

Recently I attended a day of lectures taught by traditional (allopathic) practitioners. One lecturer spent an entire morning on the treatment of canine stomach ulcers. Having left regular practice years ago and devoted myself to homeopathic medicine, I had never seen a case of ulcers, and I wondered at the amount of time and interest devoted to this topic. I quickly found out that stomach ulcers are now a significant problem in today's veterinary hospital due to the widespread use of non-steroidal-anti-inflammatories (NSAID's) such as Rimadyl, for numerous orthopedic problems. (Aspirin is also a NSAID.) Rimadyl also causes seizures, jaundice, pale gums, and coma.[7] Since NSAID's work so well to temporarily palliate lameness and other pains, their use has become widespread, and their side effects rampant, thus creating the hottest topics for continuing education courses for practicing vets. One young veterinarian expressed her dismay, wondering why we were spending so much time on a disease that could be cured by eliminating a drug. So much to tell her!

Side effects exist only when the medicine does not cover all the symptoms.

To summarize, allopathic practitioners treat functional disturbances through the administration of large doses of physiologically active substances. The medicine is given to counteract a single or small set of symptoms, and thus has many "side" effects which have no relationship to the patient's true illness. These treatments are purely palliative, in that the symptom is only temporarily mitigated, and when the medicine is discontinued, the symptom returns even stronger than before. Think of asthma medications. Once begun, the patient is hooked, because if they stop, their breathing becomes even worse than before they started the medicine! These drugs quickly become a crutch.

Homeopathy

"*The physician is likewise a preserver of health if he knows the things that disturb it, that cause and sustain illness, and if he knows how to remove them from healthy people.*"—Hahnemann, A. 4, *Organon*

Dr. Samuel Hahnemann (1755 - 1843) was a German physician who developed homeopathy into a complete system of medicine. He made homeopathy accessible in an organized, understandable, and effective manner. The term "homeopathy" is derived from the Greek words homoios pathos, meaning similar suffering.[8] The original spelling, "homœopathy," is derived from the Latin way of writing the "oi" of Greek, and was Americanized due to the difficulty of finding the proper type for the "œ."[9] Another common modern spelling is "homoeopathy," derived from the German "homöopathie." [Dr. Don Hamilton, personal communication]

Homeopathic medicines are chosen for each patient based on their similarity to the patient's disease. No symptom is left out of the disease picture, so that the matching of patient and remedy can be complete. Thus, a dog with joint pain and a history of loose foul stools will receive a different treatment than a dog with joint pain and skin eruptions. Homeopathy works within the natural laws of the body to guide the vital force out of a state of disease and into a state of health.

Homeopathic remedies treat energetic disturbances using tiny diluted doses of energetically active medicines. The proper homeopathic treatment is selected to cover all the symptoms of the case, so there are no side effects. The goal is always cure. Which would you rather have?

Law of Similars (Principle of Like Cures Like)

The Law of Similars is the foundation for homeopathy. It states that when a substance produces a symptom in a healthy person, then that same substance will treat that symptom when it naturally occurs in a sick person (or animal). The basis for the Law of Similars was known to Hippocrates in 400 B.C.[10], but much older references have been found in ancient Egyptian medical texts as well as in the *Shrimad Bhagavata Mahapurana* of India, dating from 3000 -1000 B.C. *"When a substance in its gross form produces an ailment, doesn't it refined...produce relief of the same ailment?"*[11] Thus arsenic, known to produce bloody diarrhea and vomiting, will cure this same condition, once diluted, in a patient.

Homeopathy matches all the patient's symptoms with a single medicine. This medicine cures.

Hahnemann discovered this law through meticulous, reproducible experiments, first on himself, then with a growing body of assistants. He began taking quinine, the herb used to treat malaria, after disagreeing with a medical textbook's explanation of how this herb works in the body. He found that over time, taking quinine produced in himself, a healthy person, exactly the symptoms of malaria! From this beginning, he went on to investigate the action of many other substances, thus creating a materia medica, or "body of collected knowledge about the therapeutic properties of any substance used for healing."[12] One of his works, *The Chronic Diseases: Their Peculiar Nature and Their Homoeopathic Cure*, contains timeless data that helps practitioners match remedies to patients, even in our modern world. The body does not change in how it expresses disease over generations and cultures. The respiratory system, for example, can cough or rasp or sneeze or feel heavy or produce mucus, all the same whether the patient is a peasant farmer from India or a cat in the royal family of England. From this text, a practitioner can study the symptoms produced by any homeopathic remedy, and find the image of his patient's illness in the image of the substance. This is the simillimum, or the remedy that matches the picture of the illness. Thus matched, simillimum to patient, cure follows.

Provings, or How Remedies are Known

Provings are the process by which substances are ingested daily over a few days by healthy persons, and then the body's responses are meticulously noted over time. Provings can last months, as some remedies produce symptoms for many weeks after exposure. The *Organon* provides careful instructions for conducting provings, found in aphorisms 121 — 142. (Aphorisms, designated by A., are sequentially numbered sections of the *Organon*.) "For this purpose each medicinal substance must be used completely on its own and in entirely pure form, without the admixture of any foreign substance. Nothing else of a foreign medicinal nature is to be taken on the same day nor on subsequent days for as long as one wishes to observe the effects of the medicine." (A. 124) [13] Hahnemann stresses the importance of a reliable prover in aphorism 126, saying, "The person chosen for the experiment must *above all* be *trustworthy* and *conscientious*."[14] They must also know themselves, be familiar with their body's state, and have adequate language to expresses their observations, so that they can communicate clearly and accurately the symptoms of the proving substance.

Provers are selected from a variety of different types of people. "The total picture of disease symptoms that a medicine can produce approaches completion only after multiple observations have been made on many suitable persons of both sexes, with various constitutions." (A. 135) [15] The provers must consist of a range of types, from the robust farmer to the sensitive intellectual. But all must be healthy, and able to communicate their condition faithfully and truthfully. Provings cannot be performed on non-human animals, because even though we would be able to observe some symptoms, we would only have a fragmentary image. Animals cannot communicate inner feelings and sensations clearly, or describe when exactly the symptom begins, or in what location within the body, or how their inner experience changes over time. Without their understanding and compliance, subjecting non-human animals to distressing symptoms is not only potentially misleading, but unnecessary and harsh. The essence of a good prover is the ability to communicate, making a non-human animal a poor prover indeed. Instead, we can expand our knowledge through careful clinical results on veterinary patients, proven valuable over time and with cumulative patient numbers. Meanwhile, human provings can be extrapolated carefully to the veterinary patient by experienced practitioners.

The final result of a large collection of meticulous provings is a complete picture of the substance. This is what must be matched with the patient's disease in order to cure. These symptoms are collected in books called materia medicas, which are still in use by the homeopaths of today.

• • •

Here are some more cases, to illustrate the breadth of what homeopathy can accomplish and how the treatment is selected based on the entire patient. In later chapters we will investigate case workups in greater detail.

A Dove Who Couldn't Go (reprinted with permission from the AVH—with some notations added for clarity) [16]

Wilkins, a Sacred Heart dove, was 18 years old when his guardian called me in a panic. It was a week before Christmas and I was all dressed up and ready to go out with my fiancé. Wilkins was straining and his vent (under the tail) was packed with dry hard droppings. He was depressed and his feathers were ruffled. It sounded like he might not last the night.

Bringing along my fiancé, I came to see what we could do. Along with homeopathic treatment, it seemed important to remove some of the dry hard material from his vent, but what to do with such a tiny delicate patient? His guardian handed me a tiny implement which only years later she told me was a "coke sniffing spoon." At the time, I didn't think to question it, and it filled the bill. We removed some of the built-up material and then gave him lycopodium 30X (a homeopathic remedy derived from club moss) in water, to be repeated twice daily. (30X refers to the potency, which we will discuss in later chapters.) The symptoms indicating this remedy were pretty clear: constipation, ineffectual urging and straining, inactive rectum, and pain with tenesmus (straining). Then, considering he was a bird and the material in his vent also derived from his kidneys, I included kidney inflammation, suppression of urine, and retention of urine to the mix. Then I said a short prayer and headed to the party, where I couldn't stop thinking about my patient.

Two days later, Wilkins was still straining, but only when he had a movement. His vent was still not opening or closing well, and he had a mucousy discharge with some blood. His droppings were loose (which was an improvement). He was not eating or drinking much. More history was volunteered, that he often had straining and vocalizing when having a movement. I was happy that his straining had reduced, and knowing that this was chronic disease, I did not expect a rapid recovery. Small steps. We continued the 30X lyc twice daily. One of the most difficult tasks for the homeopath is to know when to wait, when to notice the small beginnings of healing and allow the vital force to continue its work. Switching remedies at this point would have been disastrous, because the interruption of the healing changes could stop the remedy reaction permanently.

Two more days later, just before Christmas, Wilkins was still straining, but the swelling around his vent had diminished and it was now opening and closing more normally. He still had some bloody discharge and his feathers were ruffled, but he was now drinking. His feet were cold. We stopped the 30X and gave him a single dose of lycopodium 200C in a cheese ball, which he accepted readily.

By the day after Christmas, everything was back to normal. His personality had changed from distant and reserved, which he had been for his whole life, to friendly and approachable. Wilkins had responded to the remedy not only on a physical plane, but on a mental and emotional plane as well. Homeopathic treatment, based on the entire patient (not just an individual symptom), heals the entire patient, not just parts of the patient.

Wilkins received lyc 1M for similar (milder) symptoms five months later, then again another year later. After that he needed occasional doses of the same remedy, finally dying six years later at 25 years of age. A year before he died, he was still breeding.

Happily, my fiancé also survived the experience and we were married a few months later.

A Grey Squirrel with Neurological Problems (reprinted with permission from the AVH—with some notations added for clarity) [17]

This case shows that even disease present from birth can be diminished and reduced with the curative remedy. Ronnie was an elderly squirrel who didn't move around normally. She was unable to climb very well, so she had lived in captivity since birth. Recently, she had an acute onset of prostration, gasping respirations, rapid emaciation, and a greatly reduced appetite with increased thirst. This had happened before, but it had resolved without treatment. When I went to see her she was stiff and cold, even though lying on a heating pad, and she began open-mouth breathing after being handled. She could stand briefly, but only in a hunched posture, and she fell to the right.

I wanted to know what she was like before getting so desperately ill. Her guardian reported that when well, she growls when being handled. And after her bedding is changed, she avoids her box for many hours.

I began the case with arsenicum album 30X (a homeopathic remedy matched to her case—-we will discuss this matching process in later chapters), because it most closely fit her lack of appetite with thirst, her gasping respirations, her lack of vital heat, her stiffness, and her emaciation and sudden collapse. Since this problem had happened before and was now worse, I knew I was dealing with chronic disease. I did not know if she could be saved.

That evening she stopped drinking, and the following morning she had some diarrhea. She was very quiet, and did not show any improvement. Time for another remedy. I brought out lycopodium and gave it in the 30X potency, to be given three times daily. At the time I was new to homeopathy, and afraid to give higher potencies to critical cases. What drew me to this remedy was its cited helpfulness in weakening functional powers in older patients.

The following morning, Ronnie left the heating pad and grabbed food from the hands of her guardian. She was more comfortable and alert, with no further diarrhea or gasping. The remedy was discontinued. Ten days later, she was back to normal and had regained all her weight, as well as her normally irritable disposition. One month later, she was "every day a new squirrel," running all over her room and no longer tipping over. Before treatment, she had not left her shelf for the past eight months to a year. She was sleek, and held her tail in the "S" shape of a normal squirrel, which she had *never done before* in her life. She lived for another year and eight months, dying quietly in her sleep.

• • •

The advantage over modern medicines in these two cases is that they left the patients healed, without requiring lifelong or constantly repeated drugs. Also, these remedies were matched exactly to their symptoms, so that there were no side effects, which limit the usefulness of undiluted concentrated modern medications. With more experience (these cases were early in my career), the initial potency could have been higher, completely avoiding the need for daily dosing. (See the next case for an illustration of this technique.) Reducing the frequency of dosing is very helpful in birds and squirrels, as well as in many cats and dogs and people!

Chronic Weight Loss

Thomas was a 5 year-old domestic shorthair cat with severe weight loss. He had dropped from 12 lb. to 8 lb., despite high doses of steroids over the past six months. He was given a remedy based on his weight loss and his behaviors surrounding food and mealtimes. After this dose, we were able to take him off all of his allopathic medicine. He regained his normal weight of 11 lb. and he continued to do well for three more years, after which he was lost to follow-up.

As this case shows, a curative remedy does not need to be repeated. The patient is set on the right track, and the vital force does the rest. Young patients like Thomas have more vital energy to respond, and can be very rewarding patients.

A Chronic Bloody Nasal Discharge

Ida was an approximately 12 year-old female domestic shorthair cat who had been sneezing blood for the past year. By the time I saw her, she had all the symptoms of an upper respiratory tract infection. It never seemed to resolve, despite many traditional treatments. She received one dose of the homeopathic remedy which matched her entire case, and after initially worsening, all her symptoms resolved and she was "like a new cat."

This case is not typical, especially in patients who have received a lot of allopathic medications. Often these patients need repeated doses of their remedy over time before they can generate a healing response. This is because drugs given to address a single symptom, such as the antibiotics and steroids given to Ida over the past year, do not support the body's natural healing ability. Over time, the vital force weakens and the side effects, or the effects of the drug which do not match the patient, become predominant. But Ida was still strong enough to react promptly and permanently to her remedy. When the right remedy is given, the resultant healing can seem like a miracle. Energy that previously was spent producing symptoms is now freed and the patient acts younger. Older animals play again like they used to, years ago.

• • •

If these cases pique your interest and inspire you to search for a homeopathic practitioner to help your animal, then I have done my job. In the rest of the book, we will study cases in more detail to illustrate how the patient's symptoms are examined in order to match these symptoms with those of the remedy provings. But first, I will discuss how the remedies are prepared, and what exactly happens in the patient who has received a dose.

• • •

Chapter 2 References

1. Hahnemann S. *Organon of the Medical Art, Sixth Edition*. O'Reilly WB, ed. Redmond, WA: Birdcage Books;1996: 294.
2. Hahnemann S. *Organon of Medicine, Sixth Edition*. Künzli J, Naudé A, Pendleton P, eds. Blaine, WA: Cooper Publishing;1982: 71.
3. "Diabetes Mellitus." *The Merck Veterinary Manual*. Ed. David Bruyette. Merck Sharp & Dohme Corp., May 2013. Web. 5 Sept. 2015. <http://www.merckvetmanual.com/mvm/endocrine_system/the_pancreas/diabetes_mellitus.html?qt=&sc=&alt=>.
4. "Hyperthyroidism." *The Merck Veterinary Manual*. Ed. Mark E. Peterson. Merck Sharp & Dohme Corp., Aug. 2013. Web. 5 Sept. 2015.

<http://www.merckvetmanual.com/mvm/endocrine_system/the_thyroid_gland/hyperthyroidism.html?qt=hyperthyroidism&alt=sh>.

5. "Aspirin." *Drugs & Medications*. WebMD, n.d. Web. 5 Sept. 2015. <http://www.webmd.com/drugs/2/drug-1082-3/aspirin-oral/aspirin-oral/details#>.
6. *Ibid.* 1, p. 285.
7. "More Information." *Rimadyl® Caplets and Chewables (Brand).* Doctors Foster and Smith, n.d. Web. 5 Sept. 2015. <http://www.drsfostersmith.com/product/prod_display.cfm?pcatid=23266>.
8. *Ibid.* 1, p. 48.
9. Winston J. *The Faces of Homoeopathy*. Tawa, New Zealand; Great Auk Publishing; 1999: xix.
10. Close S. *The Genuis of Homoeopathy.* New Delhi, India: B. Jain Publishers;1997: 215.
11. Academic Catalogue. Blacksburg, VA: Lotus Health Institute, 2010. Homeopathic Certificate Course. Robin Murphy, N.D. Web. 3 Dec. 2012.<http://www.lotushealthinstitute.com/downloads/LHI-CourseCatalogue.pdf>.
12. "Materia Medica." *Wikipedia*. N.p., 3 Sept. 2015. Web. 5 Sept. 2015. <https://en.wikipedia.org/wiki/Materia_medica>.
13. *Ibid.* 2, p. 109.
14. *Ibid.*, p. 110.
15. *Ibid.*, p. 114.
16. Jensen W. "The Dove Who Couldn't Go." *JAcadVetHom*. Winter 1999: 3.
17. Jensen W. "Neurological Disease." *JAcadVetHom*. Winter 1999: 3.

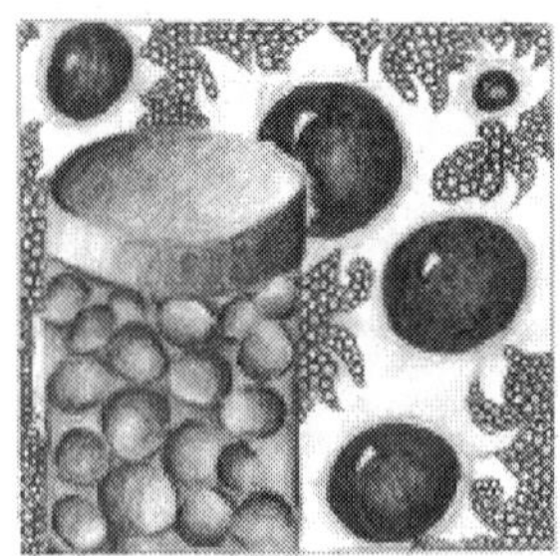

3 - The Basics

Preparation of Medicines

So what is in this medicine called homeopathy? And how is it so different from the drugs we all used as we were growing up? This chapter will explore how homeopathic remedies are made, then we will discuss what exactly happens in the patient after a dose. Your observations will help your homeopath determine how the remedy has affected your animal. This is critical information that determines the next step in treatment.

Homeopathic remedies are derived from four sources: plants, animals (insects or animal secretions such as milk or venom), minerals, and chemicals. In Boericke's *Materia Medica*, out of 554 remedies, 72% are plants, 13% are animals or animal products, and the rest are minerals or chemicals. All remedies are prepared using the same process, the only difference found at the very beginning when solid substances must be crushed and macerated (soaked in liquid) so that they can be dissolved into solution.

Remedies are substances found in nature.

The *Organon* contains strict instructions for producing homeopathic remedies, as written in A. 264 - 271. First, the fresh plant is crushed and macerated in alcohol to extract the sap, then any fibrous material is allowed to precipitate out, or sink to the bottom of the vessel, so it can be removed. This procedure allows the base material to be stored for long periods of time, if needed, without rotting or growing mold. Next, the material is thoroughly ground up and mixed with milk sugar over a period of three hours. This is called trituration and dilution, and this process serves to develop the medicinal powers of the substance. Milk sugar is used because it is quite non-reactive and has no medicinal properties of its own. Slowly, more milk sugar is added to the trituration in very specific amounts, until the original substance is diluted 1:100. This is called the one-hundredth attenuation, or first centesimal trituration, also called the 1C potency. This process of trituration and dilution is continued until the substance is diluted 1:1,000,000, or 3C. Once the remedy has reached 3C, even substances that began as solids, such as fresh plants or insects, are able to be dissolved, so that the preparation of higher potencies can continue in water and alcohol. Higher potencies are developed by repeated dilution and succussion, or shaking, all the way up to MM potencies, which is a C potency diluted and succussed one million times! A clear description of the process can be read at Hahnemann Laboratories' website.[1]

"*...homeopathy develops the inner, spirit-like medicinal powers of crude substance to a degree hitherto unheard of and makes all of them exceedingly, even immeasurably, penetrating, active, and effective, even those that in the crude state do not have the slightest medicinal effect on the human organism.*"—Hahnemann, A. 269, *Organon*

Remedies are prepared in four different potency series: X, C, M, and LM. X potencies are diluted in a ratio of 1: 10, C in a ratio of 1:100, M in a ratio of 1:1,000C, and LM in a ratio of 1:50,000. The LM's were developed by Hahnemann just before the end of his life, and they are usually administered in liquid form.

In this way, through trituration, dilution and succussion, the medicinal powers of the substance are made available to the patient. As Hahnemann writes in A. 269, "This remarkable transformation of the properties of natural bodies through the mechanical action of trituration and succussion on their tiniest particles...develops the latent *dynamic* powers previously imperceptible and as it were lying hidden asleep in them. These powers electively affect the vital principle of animal life. This process is called *dynamization* or *potentization* (development of medicinal power), and it creates what we call *dynamizations* or *potencies* of different degrees."[2]

So that's what is in those sweet-tasting little white pills—now, how do we know that anything has actually happened after the remedy is given? We are all used to judging a medicine by watching the symptoms—when the medicine is swallowed, the symptom goes away, right? But when the animal's vital force is directing the response, the game changes. We are no longer giving a strong medicine to counteract a symptom. We are stimulating the vital force to initiate healing.

Consequences of Giving a Remedy

The vital force responds in only one of three ways to any medicine:

palliation
suppression
cure

"[Palliative medicines]...spectacular for their flattering, often almost instantaneous action."—Hahnemann, A. 55, *Organon*

Palliation is the gold standard in today's modern world. We want results, and we want them now. But palliation doesn't get our animals better. "The relief is never lasting, and the symptoms always return worse than before."[3] Give Rimadyl for joint pain, and the pain eases. Give prednisone for itching, and the scratching stops. The response happens quickly, and the medicines only act upon that part of the case with matching symptoms. Rimadyl matches joint pain, and prednisone matches itching. Any medicine, remedy or pharmaceutical, can cause a palliative response.

Palliation eases symptoms, but then the symptoms rebound, and get worse over time.

Palliation is temporary. The symptoms return quickly once the medicine is discontinued, and over time and repeated doses, this recurrence happens with greater and greater intensity. Over time, the dosage must be increased in order to obtain the same relief, especially in painful conditions. Meanwhile, the duration of relief is shorter and shorter. Palliation is not a path towards cure, but simply the temporary easement of one particular symptom or symptom complex. Overall the patient is no healthier, and they continue to suffer. The vital force weakens from this treatment.

The relief caused by palliation is superficial, not able to penetrate very deeply into the economy. Read A. 23: "...persistent disease symptoms, far from being wiped out and destroyed by opposite medicinal symptoms (in the *antipathic, enantiopathic,* or *palliative method*), return instead with renewed intensity and evident aggravation after seeming for a short time to have improved."[4] This superficial change that brings only temporary relief happens quickly. This is not a slow change.

Another characteristic of a palliative prescription is that a higher potency gives even less relief than the lower potency. As in A. 60, "The orthodox physician imagines that he can get out of the difficulty by prescribing a stronger dose of the medicine with each new aggravation. This produces only another brief hushing up of the symptoms and, from the necessity to keep increasing the dose of the palliative, either some other, even worse complaint or quite often a condition of complete incurability, danger to life, even death."[5] What is Hahnemann saying? He is telling us very clearly that with repeated palliation the patient gets sicker. It's a vicious cycle, leading the practitioner on to stronger and stronger drugs even while each successive improvement is shorter.

Why do we repeat palliatives? Because they seem to help. Hahnemann writes in A. 69, "...in the first moments of the palliation the vital force feels nothing disagreeable, either from the symptom or from the opposing medicinal symptom....The vital force feels as if it were healthy...."[6] The patient looks good! The patient, briefly, feels good! We want this to happen again, and feel that more medicine is warranted. What is more powerful than this—a veritable prescription for addiction! Yet the end result is more sickness. "As in a dark dungeon, where the prisoner can only gradually and with difficulty distinguish his immediate surroundings, the sudden lighting of a lamp at once consolingly illuminates everything around him, but as soon as it is extinguished, the brighter the flame was, the darker the obscurity that follows, and the poor prisoner finds it far more difficult than before to see his surroundings."[7]

The suppressed patient, though free of symptoms, is on a path towards destruction.

Suppression is quite different, in that once the medicine is given, the symptom disappears permanently. Suppression is the forcible concealment of symptoms. If the rest of the case, including other symptoms, is not examined, this condition may be mislabeled cure, since the offending symptom has been removed. But other symptoms are unaffected or worse, and the patient is not better. The patient may look better initially, as they are no longer suffering the effects of the suppressed symptom, but there is no increase in energy or well-being, and other symptoms remain or become worse over time. It is a permanent effect, making the patient weaker. Eventually, more serious and even life-threatening symptoms arise. The disease is still present, yet driven deeper into the body, more towards vital, life-sustaining organs. As Dr. Close, an American homeopath from the 1920's writes, "Close the exhaust and an explosion follows."[8] Any medicine, including remedies, can cause suppression if given inappropriately. Suppression can also occur in patients without any medicine, whether caused by severe weather, a sudden fright, or increasing debility.

Suppression drives the illness deeper.

The goal of homeopathic treatment is cure, which is an organic event initiated by the remedy matching the entire case. The whole body is involved with a curative response. At first, it looks like nothing is happening. There's a delay while the body reacts to the healing potency. Some symptoms may even appear slightly worse, as the medicine, given for its similarity to the patient's disease, exaggerates the illness that is already present. This is called the curative aggravation. But then the magic happens. The patient appears more peaceful, calm, more "up." Enthusiasm for life returns, there is an increase in energy, animals who before were isolating now come out for some company. Over time, these changes become more pronounced, until eventually it is quite clear that something really good is happening.

Cure allows our animals to live life to the fullest.

Who does what? The impinging potence, or the medicine, causes the initial action, as in A. 63, "Every power that acts on life, every medicine, alters the vital force more or less and brings about in human health certain modifications of greater or less duration. We call this the *primary action*."[9] Then the vital force reacts to this impingement, or primary action, by a counter-action, or secondary action, which reduces the disease load in the body. From A. 69: "...the secondary action is...the counteraction of the vital force."[10] The remedy starts the process, and the body completes it. Healing is only achieved when the vital force is an active participant.

The strength of the curative remedy has been likened to that of the sun. Imagine a candle burning in a dark room. Fairly illuminating, yes? But once the sun rises, the light from the candle fades to almost nothing by comparison. Thus the strength of the disease (the candle) is nothing compared to the deep down curative counter-action of the vital principle, stimulated by the remedy.

During the course of the illness, curative remedies often cause old unresolved symptoms to return. This is a very good sign that the vital force is getting down to some really deep housecleaning. Cure may be initiated by the remedy, but it is maintained strictly by the vital force. It is an ongoing process that brings our animals back to life.

• • •

So now we know what is being treated in our animals, how homeopathy works, how remedies are made, and what happens after the administration of a remedy. Now let's get into the process of remedy selection and case management. "Why study more?" you might ask. If you understand the steps taken by your homeopath to select and treat chronic disease, then you will be a more effective participant in your animal's care. As veterinarians treating non-speaking patients, we are dependent upon you to give us the best information possible before we can even begin to consider the proper treatment. You are your animal's best advocate and also the person who knows them, inside and out. If you also understand what information your vet needs and how they work to select the best treatment, you will be able to provide the most competent and effective help possible for your loved one's return to health. This is where the fun begins! But first, here are two more cases to illustrate success even in the face of very serious illness. The first case shows how homeopathy can be effective even in the midst of traditional medications.

Feline Urinary Blockage

Solly was five years old, a domestic short-hair cat, when he was discovered out on his driveway (his favorite place to hang out), weak and sick. This was August of 2006. He had had a little cough that morning, and wouldn't drink. He had been outside all day. Fearing trauma, I recommended a quick visit to the veterinary hospital. (Solly lived far away so I was not able to see him in my own hospital.) His urethra was completely blocked and he was unable to pass urine.

This blocked condition is an emergency. Since Solly typically urinates outside rather than in a cat box in the house, his condition had gone unnoticed until he was nearly comatose. He needed urgent life-saving care before he could return home and receive homeopathic treatment. If he had been able to come to my hospital, I could have unblocked him there and proceeded with homeopathic care, but his only option was a traditional hospital, in order to save his life.

I was very concerned about Solly, because of the severity and suddenness of his symptoms. Usually, the course of this disease begins with episodes of straining and bloody urine, often spontaneously resolving before the patient cycles back into gradually worsening attacks. Finally, after many such episodes, the patient may block completely, necessitating a rush to the veterinarian for catheterization of the urethra and sometimes surgery to remove the narrowed portion of the urethra. Solly had never experienced these early obvious attacks—instead, he went right into the emergency state of blockage. His vital force was very weak.

• • •

Upon admittance to the allopathic emergency hospital, Solly was catheterized to allow him to urinate, and blood work was performed. His kidney function values were elevated four times above normal, indicating that these organs were not working well. Three days later, after fluid treatment, his values had reduced to only twice the normal levels. This showed that his kidneys were responding to the removal of the blockage, and that the damage was potentially reversible. Good news! Finally, his catheter was removed and he was able to urinate on his own. Solly was sent home.

At home, he was not himself. He didn't want to be picked up or touched, and he didn't want to be on the bed. "Everything is so slow with Solly. He walks, 'Thud, thud.'" He wouldn't move off the driveway even if a car was coming. He was losing a lot of fur, and had a fair amount of white dander.

The main goal of treatment now was to avoid a repeat blockage, which is common in male cats. With homeopathy, I can treat his *tendency* to get blocked, instead of waiting until he blocks again. In addition, not only will he heal faster from this current condition, but future recurrences will be less severe and less frequent, until finally he stops having urinary troubles at all. Homeopathy reverses the normal progression of chronic disease.

The difficulty with urinary blockages is that the symptoms are often very common, thus not pointing to a particular remedy. (See the chapter Case Analysis for a discussion of the symptoms that point to the curative remedy.) This makes it even more important to look at Solly's whole case in order to determine what remedy is the best for him. Luckily, there are concomitant symptoms (symptoms happening at the same time) which characterize Solly's case more closely. He had a cough. He was desperately afraid of thunderstorms, running to hide in the garage, and becoming "almost catatonic." This last symptom was new, making it even more useful to characterize his current state. My client noted that he doesn't meet his family's eyes when they interact with him (this is not new), and they called him "sweet but not snuggly." Also, his urine had been very bloody in the hospital.

Overall, Solly was unreactive. He was unreactive to the blockage (he was never seen trying to urinate), to the treatment, and to being home again. So after preparing his timeline and his symptom list (as in the chapter The Intake Consultation), I studied his case and found sulfur (also spelled sulphur) was the best match. Not only did it fit Solly's symptoms, but this remedy is known to help patients who are stalled, not responding to anything. I prescribed sulfur 30X, which was the potency on hand, and had my client pick up sulfur 30C (a higher potency) to hold.

• • •

After studying the case, homeopaths select the remedy which matches the symptoms most closely. This is done by using a reference text called a repertory, which indexes all the possible disease symptoms and lists remedies found in each. Many practitioners have repertories in a computer program, which makes the work much less time-consuming. After selecting a list of possible remedies, homeopaths then turn to the materia medica to verify their choices. Materia medicas are textbooks or computer programs which contain incredibly detailed descriptions of the symptoms of each remedy. Some materia medicas organize symptoms according to the location in the body, others have all the symptoms grouped together in one listing for each remedy. Here are selections from various materia medicas describing sulfur symptoms. Look at how closely each selection portrays Solly's illness:

sulfur:
[W]ill not be looked at....[11]
Urinary Organs: Retention of urine....discharge of bloody urine....[12]
Nervous System: Feels tired and used up; not rested in morning...Lassitude:

> in morning; in evening; after walking, with sleepiness. Weakness: after a short walk; after a stool; in afternoon. Exhaustion of whole body; extreme faintness; uneasiness.[13]

...is always worse before a storm.[14]

The remedy sulfur has Solly's dislike of being looked at, along with his tiredness, the plodding, and his lack of reaction. Also, sulfur patients are aggravated before a storm, which certainly fits Solly's fear. What aggravates a mental symptom is very helpful in narrowing remedy choices. (For a discussion of aggravations, see the chapter on Case Analysis, under "Modalities.")

• • •

In addition to antibiotics from the emergency veterinarian, Solly was on phenoxybenzamine, which helps the urethra relax. (Single-symptom therapy.) My job was to slowly get him off his traditional meds so that he could free up enough energy to react to his homeopathic remedy. That evening Solly was still groggy, so the guardian gave him sulfur 30C. After his dose, he relaxed and purred and ate dinner "with gusto." However, two days later he was straining to urinate, and shaking his tail in irritation. Though distressing, this was an improvement in his overall vitality. He was now reacting strongly and obviously to his urinary condition, rather than simply lying down and preparing to die. I checked the materia medica for sulfur again, to be sure these new symptoms were present, and here they are, indicating that this remedy still fits Solly:

Urinary Organs: Frequent urging to urinate, but only a few drops are discharged...urine escapes slowly in drops from urethra; pains continue after urination....Constant painful urging to urinate, with frequent discharge of a few drops of urine....[15]

• • •

I advised that Solly return to his local veterinarian, to assure that he was not blocking again. On the way, he urinated on his guardian's lap. This meant that he was not blocked. Emergency averted! Nevertheless, the doctor prescribed Valium (a sedative and muscle relaxant to help the muscles in his urethra relax) and Tagamet (to reduce a presumed increase in stomach acid which can be a problem in kidney disease). This veterinarian was doing the best medicine she knew, just like I would have done before learning homeopathy, treating each symptom with its own medication. She had not been trained to treat the inner imbalance causing his disease.

The client took him home and called me. We stopped the phenoxy, put aside the Valium and Tagamet, and just waited. There was evidence that the sulfur was still helping, as shown by his irritation, his straining (new for this bout!), and his ability to urinate. His vital force had come alive and he was finally reacting! That evening he did look more comfortable, and he was more social. Solly was beginning to come out of the fog of medications. However, a urine test showed that his kidneys were still spilling protein, indicating that their ability to retain this important nutrient was still compromised.

Six days later, he was still having straining episodes, leaving little spots of urine all over the house. Instead of blocking and entering a near-comatose state, though, he was reacting to his disease with non-life-threatening local inflammation. He was struggling to heal, but he needed more time for his weakened vital force to recover. I sent sulfur LM1, to hold. But he didn't need it. In two more days, he was much better, visiting his family in bed in the mornings, ready to eat, and being his companionable self. His blood values had also improved. Over the next couple of months, he was generally well, with occasional bouts of vomiting and hunger so excessive he would bite his person in the morning until she fed him! His urine got more concentrated, back to what is normal for cats, and his kidneys were no longer spilling protein. Eventually his blood work values returned to near normal.

Over the next several months, I put Solly's person on high alert, so that we wouldn't miss any hint of trouble. In December we repeated the sulfur 30C, then giving sulfur 200C when he showed increased thirst, was sleeping more, and again not wanting to be stroked or handled at all. At this time his fur was also "lank," and he was hiding. The same remedy turned him around each time. Solly eventually recovered fully, "Sprinting up the driveway, tail high!"

Solly lived another six years and seven months, receiving infrequent doses of his remedy when he needed it, but he never blocked again. He was euthanized at age twelve after a sudden illness that progressed rapidly, with no definitive diagnosis. At that time his kidney levels were "not too bad," in spite of severe dehydration. When it is their time to go, sometimes patients treated with homeopathy move more quickly through the dying process. Without an autopsy, we don't have a sure cause of death for Solly. However, until the end, he remained entirely free of urinary tract disease. He continued to be worried about thunderstorms, but was more calm than before homeopathic treatment. As his guardian said of her beloved cat, "He had a much healthier and longer life with your excellent care."

• • •

The sooner you remove obstacles to cure (suppressive medications) the sooner cure can happen. The vital force can only react as a unit. So if unsuitable medications are administered, the vital force is busy trying to react, changing under pressure, producing some new symptoms related to the drug (side effects), and generally changing its state from what it was prior to the drugs. This change of state is not necessarily in a good direction. Hahnemann writes about drugs prescribed based on single symptoms, "Incomparably more frequent than natural dissimilar diseases associating and complicating themselves in the same body are those disease complications that the inexpedient medical procedure (the allopathic mode of treatment) tends to bring to pass through the protracted use of unsuitable medicines. As a result of the persistent repetition of unfitting medicines, new, often very protracted disease states (corresponding to the nature of the allopathic medicines) associate themselves to the natural disease to be cured. These new disease states gradually pair up and complicate themselves with the dissimilar chronic malady that the unsuitable medicines could not cure....In this way, a new, dissimilar, artificial chronic disease is added to the old natural disease, thus making the hitherto simply diseased individual doubly diseased, that is, much more diseased and more incurable, sometimes even entirely incurable. This double disease often kills."[16] When a single symptom is opposed (such as with Valium and Tagamet), the body reacts by trying to produce that symptom even more powerfully, or if the vital force is too weak, another more serious symptom is produced in its stead. Then another drug is prescribed for the new symptom. This eventually weakens the vital force so much that it can no longer maintain equilibrium. In Solly's case, death was close.

• • •

Here's another case that intermixes conventional medicine and homeopathy. This mixing situation might come up for you with your own animals, since we don't yet have many full-service homeopathic veterinary hospitals available to care for our animal's critical care and surgical needs. This case describes the use of homeopathy after surgery, when the patient has not rallied as expected.

The Dog Who Ate A Walnut

Ruthie is a five year-old Airedale who presented to me nine days after she had surgery to remove a walnut obstructing her intestine. She had been fine until a week after her surgery, when she developed a fever, cough and abdominal tenderness. She had not had a bowel movement for the past nine days! This is an indication of ileus, or a paralysis of the intestines. Luckily, Ruthie had other symptoms which helped characterize her disease state.

Ruthie's symptom list (we will discuss the development of the symptom list in the chapter The Intake Consultation):

post-surgical, foreign body obstruction
fever with cough and belly tenderness

lethargy
anorexia
no bowel movement for nine days (ileus)

In Ruthie's case, her two most unusual symptoms are ileus, and having a cough during a fever. They are the most descriptive of Ruthie's case. Ileus is the most uncomfortable symptom, the one of most concern, and also the one that could be the source of much of the other symptoms. It's normal to have lethargy after surgery, especially when the bowels have not yet recovered. It's also normal to have pain in the abdomen after surgery. If this pain was striking in some way, to make it stand out, then it might be a good symptom to point to a remedy. For example, if Ruthie was moving differently because of the pain, growling when anyone came near, or trying to have a bowel movement but stopping with a shriek because of the pain, then the pain would be more central to her case.

The remedy that fit all of her symptoms most closely was phosphorus. Here is how phosphorus reads in the materia medica:

phosphorus:
Fever: ...with oppression of chest and difficult respiration...racking cough with thick, yellow or reddish expectoration...threatened paralysis of lungs; coma, with hot breath and rattling, as if a large quantity of phlegm were rattling in lungs....[17]
Abdomen: Peritonitis with tympanitis [gaseous distention]; abdomen excessively sensitive to touch...sharp cutting pains; paralysis of intestines.[18]
Boericke: ...post-operative vomiting....[19] (This was important to note because even though Ruthie was not vomiting, her symptoms were occurring in the post-operative state.)
Allen: Paralysis of the intestines.[20]

Some symptoms in the materia medica are from cured cases, mixed in with the proving symptoms, as discussed in the chapter What Does Homeopathy Heal? When the remedy has repeatedly shown itself useful in practice, the symptoms of the cured patient are added to the remedy. This information would enrich veterinary materia medicas, instead of potentially misleading and inhumane animal provings. For example, "post-operative vomiting," was added by Boericke to his materia medica when he found it helpful for this condition. This greatly expands the usefulness of the materia medica, because often our patients have more severe symptoms than would be seen in a proving.

• • •

Phosphorus relates to Ruthie's suffering most closely. So that is the remedy that she needed. I prescribed phosphorus 30C, a single dose, and within a half hour, she began moving around. She went out in the yard, had a normal bowel movement, and then she ate. Three months later I received a note, "Has not stopped since magic white pills given!"

Phosphorus helps with foreign bodies associated with tenderness of the abdomen. We don't know if she had another problem that was not found at surgery, or if her body was unable to heal in spite of the surgery and the damage caused by the walnut remained, but it was the right remedy for Ruthie!

• • •

Chapter 3 References

1. "FAQs for the Hahnemann Pharmacy Web Site." Hahnemann Laboratories, Inc., n.d. Web. 5 Sept. 2015. <http://www.hahnemannlabs.com/faq.html>.
2. Hahnemann S. *Organon of Medicine, Sixth Edition.* Künzli J, Naudé A, Pendleton P, eds. Blaine, WA: Cooper Publishing;1982: 188.
3. *Ibid.*, p. 58.
4. *Ibid.*, p. 26.
5. *Ibid.*, p. 58.
6. *Ibid.*, p. 66.

7. *Ibid.*, p. 68.
8. Close S. *The Genuis of Homoeopathy.* New Delhi, India: B. Jain Publishers;1997: 75.
9. *Ibid.* 2, p. 62.
10. *Ibid.*, p. 68.
11. Hering C. *The Guiding Symptoms of Our Materia Medica.* Vol. 10. Paharganj, New Delhi, India: B. Jain Publishers;1995: 179.
12. *Ibid.*, p. 136.
13. *Ibid.*, p. 159
14. Clarke JH. *Dictionary of Practical Materia Medica* from *ReferenceWorks.* [computer program] Version 2.6.6. San Rafael, CA: Kent Homeopathic Associates.
15. *Ibid.* 11, p. 137.
16. Hahnemann S. *Organon of the Medical Art, Sixth Edition.* O'Reilly WB, ed. Redmond, WA: Birdcage Books;1996: 87-88.
17. *Ibid.* 11 (Vol. 8), p. 383.
18. *Ibid.*, p. 349.
19. Boericke W. *Materia Medica with Repertory.* Santa Rosa, CA: Boericke & Tafel, Inc.; 1927: 408.
20. Allen TF. *The Encyclopedia of Pure Materia Medica: A Record of the Positive Effects of Drugs Upon the Healthy Human Organism.* from *ReferenceWorks.* [computer program] Version 2.6.6. San Rafael, CA: Kent Homeopathic Associates.

4 - The Intake Consultation and Development of the Patient Record

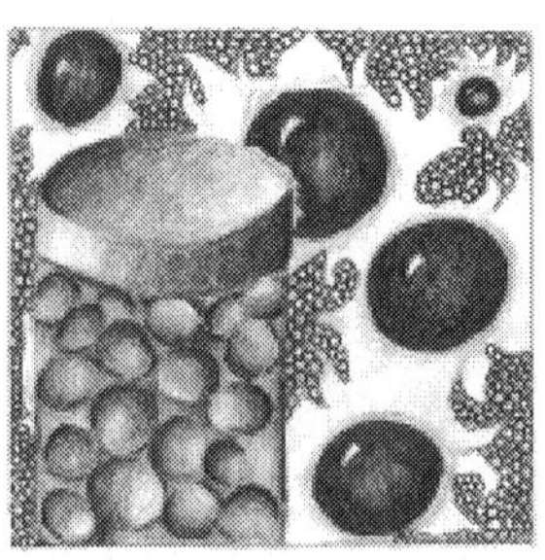

"Stories shift their shape, change character, take on different colors depending on the words you use, the language in which you choose to tell them. Sometimes more serious, sometimes more playful, more melodic, say...." [1]

The intake consultation introduces your animal to your veterinary homeopath. You are familiar with office appointments, usually scheduled into ten- or fifteen- minute slots, during which you discuss your animal's symptoms, followed by a thorough examination. Homeopathic intake consultations are quite different. During these appointments, you will share everything you know about your animal. This conversation with your veterinarian, called "taking the case," will cover all aspects of the patient, from personality quirks to physical complaints to illnesses way back in puppy- or kittenhood. How does your animal change when the weather changes? What happens when guests come over? In the case of horses, how does she behave in the show ring? What about when the farrier comes? What kinds of treatments did he receive for that chronic cough? How about his appetite? How does she get along with other animals? or people? What did last year's ear discharge look like, and smell like?

The intake consultation is a wonderful chance to share everything you know about your companion with someone who cares deeply about every detail. This may take an hour or more, unless your animal is quite young. During this appointment, your homeopath will take copious notes, listening carefully and only asking questions to fill in the blanks, or to cover areas you may not think to mention. What they are doing is learning about your animal from the inside out, so that they have the complete picture of who he really is. Without knowing the patient, the homeopath cannot select the proper treatment. Successful prescribing rests on the foundation of a well-taken case.

This chapter will give examples of good case-taking, so that you will know what to expect from your intake interview. We will also discuss how your vet will process the resultant data, preparatory to determining the correct remedy. By understanding how the intake consult information is employed, you will have a greater appreciation for the importance of a quality interview. Nowadays, virtually every veterinary homeopath began life as a traditional practitioner, taught over years of study to treat the symptoms apart from the patient. We are all, vets and clients, learning to re-educate ourselves to focus instead on the patient as a whole. The more you as a client understand what it means to take a good case, the better the case will be.

A well-informed client is one of the best friends of the veterinary homeopath.

Components of a Complete Case

intake interview
timeline
symptom list

What is the purpose of the intake interview? To get the "picture" of the patient. This is the data the veterinary homeopath needs in order to match patient to treatment. As homeopaths, we don't use blood work or X-ray images or even diagnostic labels to determine the proper remedy for a patient. We treat based on how the individual patient reacts to their own unique illness. The patient reaction is told by their symptoms.

Laboratory values, while helpful in order to determine the prognosis, are absolutely useless as a guide to treatment.

After the patient returns home, the real work begins in the homeopath's office. Studying the data from the interview, along with the physical examination results, and also any past health records, including diagnostics, your homeopath then proceeds to develop your companion's timeline and symptom list. Together the interview, timeline, and symptom list make up the triad of a complete case. Just as one cannot expect a bountiful harvest from poor seeds, neither can prescriptions be accurate with incomplete case notes and truncated (or missing!) timelines or symptom lists. Time taken early in the case will save time later, as the selected remedies will be more correct, and your animal will improve more quickly.

The timeline, the second leg of a great case, allows your homeopath to rapidly evaluate whether a particular symptom is historical, current yet longstanding, or of recent origin. Differentiation between old and new symptoms is crucial, because when old symptoms come back during homeopathic treatment, that's a very good sign. New symptoms, on the other hand, may occur when chronic disease is progressing in spite of treatment, or when the potency of a helpful remedy is incorrect. Therefore, knowing the difference between an old and a new symptom is quite important in determining the next step in treatment. I will discuss the timeline in more detail later in the chapter, together with examples from real patients. We will examine how patients often heal in the reverse order from which they became ill. Take the case of a dog who had skin eruptions, which then disappeared before he developed diarrhea, at which point he was brought in for homeopathic veterinary care. This dog will show an improvement in his diarrhea first, then he may break out in the same type of skin eruptions he used to get in the past, all in the course of healing.

The third leg of the well-taken case is the symptom list. A meticulously-crafted symptom list ensures that nothing is missed or forgotten during follow-up appointments. Often improvements in symptoms are subtle, and easily missed in the beginning. (Remember the difference between palliation and cure?) A good practitioner will check in periodically about every symptom, to understand how the whole patient is doing. Subtle improvements to a number of symptoms is just as good, if not better, than a dramatic improvement in only one symptom. Vet and client cannot risk focusing on one symptom, or the case will become derailed. Treating the patient based on one (however serious) symptom is reverting back to allopathic, or symptom-based practice, and will not produce the desired results. The patient gets better only as a whole, so all symptoms must be evaluated regularly, even old symptoms that have not recurred in years. Only when the entire patient is both matched with the proper remedy and monitored for progress, only then will you and your vet achieve the best possible results. Not every patient can be saved, but for the best chance of a good outcome, always keep the whole animal in view.

Many clients want to have a symptom list of their own, so they know what to monitor. Opinions differ on this practice, but I find it more worthwhile to have a report based on what my clients observe, rather than checking off items on a list. This way, again, the patient is looked at as a whole, not as a collection of symptoms. For example, I may be wanting to hear about their bowel habits and appetite, but more importantly, how is she feeling? Was there a lightness in her eyes that wasn't there before the prescription? Did she come running to greet you whereas before she continued her nap on the couch when you got home? If my client is following a list, I have artificially narrowed their observations to areas that may be important but don't necessarily give me the whole picture. So report what you see and feel. If your homeopath needs more information after you have given your report, they will ask the necessary questions.

Intake Interview

As if watching a flower unfold, each petal curling out to catch the sun's rays and settle into its perfect state of beauty, thus does the interview have its own pace, its own internal design. As veterinarians, we see our patients through the eyes of those closest to them. This vantage point is unique among medical professionals, with the exception of those treating babies, or humans without language due to a severe illness or disability. As veterinary homeopaths, we must above all listen, and meanwhile gently and unobtrusively maintain the focus of the conversation on fruitful ground. We want our clients to be storytellers.

A good homeopath wants to know what you know about your animal.

Don't expect your veterinarian to do much of the talking. He wants to hear your story, your "picture," as it were, of the patient. From the footnote to A. 84 in the *Organon*: "Every interruption disturbs the speakers' train of thought, and afterward they cannot remember exactly what they wanted to say."[2] The storytelling mind has a natural flow from one picture to another, curving around to connect important landmarks. If left undisturbed, the key information will float up into view.

A good homeopath will wait for your story to come to its natural end before interrupting. When the flow has finished and your story has wound down, only then does she step out of her silent listening mode to ask a few non-directed questions. Non-directed, or open-ended questions are those that cannot be answered with a "yes" or "no." Even though delicate questions might bring out more useful points and fill out details, your homeopath can never ask enough questions to fill in an unfinished story. Our animals (and ourselves!) are just too complex to be filled in like blanks on a form. One of the more delightful bits of story I received recently (without asking a question) was that my patient, a little dog, would calm down dramatically when the piano was played. And then he would sing along!

As Dr. Close says in *The Genius of Homoeopathy*, "It is a good rule to keep the patient talking, but say little yourself during an examination; to let him tell his story in his own way, without interruption, except to bring him back to the subject if he digresses. We may start him in his narrative by asking when and how his trouble began, and we may instruct him to be as definite as possible in relating his history and in locating and describing his sensations *as they seem to him*. We should not laugh at him nor pedantically correct his errors. We should not ask 'leading questions,' nor 'put words in his mouth,' but let him express his feelings and observations in his own way."[3] The same wise words apply to your homeopath's interview. You, the one most connected to the animal, must be allowed to talk freely, unmolested, so that the clearest picture can emerge, free of the homeopath's influence. More wise words from Hahnemann: "Thus the physician elicits further particulars about each of the patient's statements without ever putting words into his mouth or asking a question that can be answered only by yes or no, which induces the patient to affirm something untrue or half true or else deny something really there to avoid discomfort or out of desire to please, thereby giving a wrong picture of the disease, which would lead to the wrong treatment."[4] (Hahnemann treated humans, but his words, as quoted throughout this book, apply equally well to the animal patient, or to the person speaking for the patient.)

Dr. Alain Naudé, editor of the *Organon*, informed me that laziness is the key to taking the best case. In other words, your homeopath will do best to *just listen*. A. 83: "This individualizing *examination of a case of disease*...demands of the physician only impartiality, sound senses, attentive observation, and faithfulness in recording the disease picture."[5]

• • •

Here's the first part of one interview from my practice, written as much as possible word for word. As you read through it, notice how the initial seemingly digressing tangents actually serve to shake out all the important facets of the case. The client's words are in quotes, and my thoughts are in square brackets. Hogarth is a seven year-old neutered male Labrador Retriever dog, with a persistent bloody nasal discharge in spite of multiple courses of antibiotics and anti-fungal medications.

• • •

Client: "Three months ago Hogarth began sneezing. There also was a gucky discharge. Recently it's become all blood, all over the carpet. Like someone had a knife and it wasn't Hogarth!"

WJ: [Such a vivid description! The case immediately comes alive for us.]

Client: "X-rays showed no tumor, just cloudiness on the right side of the nasal cavity. Awhile ago he did get some porcupine quills in his nose, and we pulled them out ourselves."

WJ: [My ears pricked up here, because an embedded porcupine quill could be causing the bleeding. But interrupting now will change the client's focus to a past event instead of the patient as he is now. I am not trying to determine the cause of this one symptom, but rather trying to see the patient as a whole. So I'll simply make a note to ask later when this occurred, and consider at that time whether additional diagnostics might be helpful to rule out the presence of a quill.]

Client: "In the past month he began gurgling with his breathing, and now it's happening even at night."

WJ: [Very helpful timeline information. Many of us don't retain such a clear presentation of the sequence of events. This clearly delineates the progression of chronic disease in this patient, so we can tell how fast things are changing.]

Client: "Now his discharge is bloody, and out of both nostrils."

WJ: [I make a note to ask which nostril was first, because the side of the body is important in homeopathy.]

Client: "About 1½ months ago his nose got dry. He's always been fearful of loud noises. At first the discharge was only on the right side."

WJ: [Ah! Question answered and no interruption to the flow of the client's memory.]

Client: "Last month he had no bloody vent until yesterday."

WJ: [This is a period of 3½ weeks. So now we have a frequency for the bloody blow-outs. Frequencies are essential for proper follow-ups, because they help your vet properly evaluate the effectiveness of the treatment.]

Client: "He was maybe better on anti-fungals, but he's not better now. Here's the medication he has been on." (She shows me a bottle of Rimadyl.)

• • •

Since she slowed down and stopped here, I took the opportunity to ask about this medication. It might indicate other symptoms that she hadn't yet talked about, since it is often used to ease lameness in older dogs.

Client: "Oh yeah, he was on it for his arthritis."

WJ: "How does he show his arthritis?" [Notice this is a non-directed question, without a "yes" or "no" answer.]

Client: "One morning he was just laying, moaning. It was hard for him to get up his hindquarters. He had to be carried down the stairs in the morning. It went away after two doses....At first the discharge was watery blood, and it's been bad at least three times. Bad blow-outs. He's a protective dog, loyal especially to Dad. He stays by Dad."

WJ: "How else does he show this loyalty?" [To get more details without assuming anything.]

Client: "He might react to say men coming out of a crummy truck. One day [the client's son] was with him out in the yard and a man got out of his truck and Hogarth growled and attacked. He has bit, nipped a couple of people when they came near the kids, very protective, but he's never broken skin. He's the enforcer, whereas Rorie [the other dog] rings the bell [gets everybody going]. He's got a good temperament. Through all this he eats. He occasionally skips [eating], like always."

• • •

Once the patient's story is done, then and only then comes the time for questions. I now go back over what has already been said, so that each point is recorded clearly and completely. I fill in details wherever possible, such as the quality of the discharges, what makes each symptom worse or better (these are symptom modalities which will be covered in the chapter Case Analysis), what symptoms occur at the same time as other symptoms (these are called concomitant symptoms), and how each particular symptom affects the overall well-being of the patient. Symptoms that bother the patient are usually more important in the case.

A good interviewer is not afraid to ask questions. Here Dr. Close describes overcoming his own modesty in order to get at the facts, when interviewing a patient with tuberculosis (called phthisis pulmonalis in the old texts): "I often recall with amusement my feelings as I witnessed for the first time an examination of a case of phthisis pulmonalis by my old preceptor, Dr. Wells. The part of the examination which excited my risibilities [tendency to laugh] was that which referred to the character of the sputum [coughed up mucus]. He inquired particularly as to its color, *odor*, form and *taste*! It was the first time I had ever heard such questions and the first time that it had ever been brought home to me that such facts could have any bearing upon the selection of the remedy."[6]

• • •

It's now time for me to direct the course of the interview. As written in A. 86, "When the speakers have finished what they wanted to say, the physician adds to each individual symptom more precise information by questioning...."[7] Now I begin filling out the details of what has already been revealed. This part of the interview can be frustrating to the client, as they may have forgotten the details of their animal's symptoms. If this happens to you, just know that you are not alone. If you don't know the answer to a question, just say so. Anything you remember will be helpful.

So let's get back to Hogarth. (Some questions and answers are left out due to negative responses.)

WJ: "When did Hogarth get hit by the porcupine?" and "When did the arthritis begin?" and "What else did he have trouble with when suffering with his arthritis?" (Of course, there are pauses between each question to allow for the answer.)

Client: "When he began having trouble with his arthritis, he had trouble going down stairs."

WJ: "How was it for him going up the stairs?" and "What kind of noises bother him and what exactly does he do when frightened in this way?" and "What exactly was his nasal discharge like when it first started?"

Client: "A greenish cloudy goo."

WJ: [This is interesting, because when the client came to me it was for Hogarth's bloody nasal discharge. It's very helpful to know that things were different in the beginning. Often the early presentation of a symptom is more specific to the proper remedy than the later evolution of the symptom. Now I might ask how the discharge changed over time, and when did these changes happen? When was he taking the Rimadyl? When was he on the anti-fungal medications? How were his symptoms affected by each medication? And finally, when were the last doses given of each medication?]

. . .

See how each question ferrets out missing pieces of data? We aren't going somewhere new, only revisiting what has already been said in order to complete the picture, as much as is possible. Here are some questions that your homeopath might ask in order to fill out the data you have already provided (taken from A. 89 of the *Organon*): "How often does this or that complaint occur, and what brings it on each time? Does it occur while sitting, lying, standing, moving? Only on an empty stomach, or at least in the morning, or only in the evening, or only after eating—or when?"[8] See how these questions draw out information? None of them can be answered with a yes or no. The details are sometimes elusive, but an experienced homeopath will help you remember.

Details are gold to the homeopath.

Now that Hogarth's story has been told, and all the details fully understood and acknowledged, I explore other areas not covered in the initial interview. Like a spiral, every time a new symptom is discovered, I listen first and then direct questions so that the case information is completely explored.

WJ: "Where did you get him?"

Client: "From the pound. His previous owner had died, and the son's girlfriend brought him in."

WJ: "Has he had any other illnesses?"

Client: "He's never been sickly, even now. He snores at night since he's been ill. He's a good water dog, always the first in the water. He's good at getting the stick. We call him Eeyore. He lets the kids dress him up. He gets along perfectly with Rorie, right away. He may growl if excited by someone at the door, but he doesn't get upset if Rorie pushes him around."

WJ: "How does he sleep?"

Client: "Sometimes he has to potty in the middle of the night. He messed in the house only one or two times, rarely. He has large kidneys."

WJ: "How is his thirst?"

Client: "Normal."

Often a homeopath will ask you what you mean by "normal." This is not a challenge, but rather an effort to clarify. My definition of "normal" thirst might be very different from your definition of "normal" thirst. It's not about who is right, but rather an effort to find out exactly what the patient is doing. Clarity demands avoiding assumptions.

Client: "He drinks all the time, no matter the temperature of the water."

WJ: "How is he affected by different weather?"

Client: "He doesn't like to go out in the rain, but he will. Before the arthritis started, at times he had to be carried downstairs. He had a hard time especially coming down the stairs. A hard time getting his hindquarters up in the mornings. Now he comes right down."

WJ: [I make a note here to tell her that this suppressed symptom might recur during the course of treatment.]

Client: "Where we used to live he had five acres to roam, but he didn't go off by himself. He did always dig out of the chain link fence, and once he even cut his back on the fence. Houdini. Then he would sit on the porch. He didn't want to leave your side."

WJ: "How did he handle the move to this house?"

Client: "Fine, he had a good time."

WJ: "Does he have a favorite food?"

Client: "None."

WJ: "Does he have any problems with his ears and eyes?"

Client: "No."

WJ: [Oops, you can see that I asked a couple of "yes or no" questions, and that I got very little in return. Better: "How have his eyes and ears been?" and "What are his favorite foods?" I can always come back to that.]

Client: "His breath smells, we have noticed this quite a few times."

WJ: "How is his digestion?"

Client: "He will vomit up pieces of rabbits when he used to steal them from the cat at our other house. He gets along with the cat, and will chase him in play if he is told to."

WJ: "How's his skin and coat?"

Client: "He has heavy heavy shedding, more in the spring, but there is always hair all over the house, dust bunnies. He has no dandruff. When he is outside his nose is on the ground, sniffing every place."

WJ: [Do you see how some things come out as more important to the case, such as shedding in this patient? This was revealed naturally, not woodenly from a one-size-fits-all questionnaire. Dust bunnies. What vivid language!]

See how I'm traveling around the body, as organized as a physical examination? Systematic. I explore sleep, thirst and appetite, odors, training experiences, reactions to different weather, events such as coughing, sneezing, vomiting, or diarrhea, behavior with children and strangers, as well as all the body parts and functions (eyes, ears, nose, teeth and gums, breath, respiration, digestion, stool, urination, skin and coat, anal glands, gait, also feet and nails). I also always ask about general energy levels and activity, how the dog enjoys walks or car rides, how they respond to other animals or to discipline, whether the cat has been declawed or not, and how they spend their time when alone. If you are interested in other possible areas that your homeopath might explore, read the footnotes to aphorisms 88 and 89 for more suggestions: "What about going to stool?...What about sleep, during the daytime, at night?...What is the appetite like, and the thirst? How does he feel after eating or drinking?"[9]

Client: "At first he was not bad at night, he'd sneeze and a little would come out. No skin stuff, no bumps or warts. He's on tick stuff."

WJ: "Does he prefer hotter or cooler weather?"

Client: "He has no preference for any particular weather temperatures. But he does like to be next to the wood stove, definitely."

WJ: "How does he do with training?"

Client: "He is very obedient unless it's about barking, or unless he's outside. He learned to flip treats off his nose, and he can catch flies! The only dog I ever knew who can do that."

The intake interview is complete! Hogarth's story was relayed without interruption, the details filled in, and then the last missing pieces of the puzzle were discovered. Now it's time for a physical examination, from head to tail. All during the interview, I noted Hogarth's attitude and behavior as well. Another advantage of a long office visit is that even the most nervous patient may relax considerably and reveal how he reacts to sounds, smells, and the boredom of a long wait. Horses may even fall asleep in their cross ties!

It's a flow, different for everyone, but each shares a similarity of process. Just like the limbs of a tree, each interview is unique, but all have the same branching pattern and general overall shape. At the beginning, you are probably eager to talk about your animal's main symptom, which is the reason you sought help in the first place. Then, like the sprouting of limbs and the emergence of leaves, the rest of the case unfolds. Your interviewer will take the time to listen. He won't fill up silences right away, because silences allow you to compose your mind and prepare the next bit of information. Not every space has to be filled with conversation. Silences give memories space to emerge. If *allowed* rather than *directed*, memories most easily lift to the surface. The examiner's questions most beneficially come only after the client's flow slows. This moment might come fairly soon with the reserved person, or much later with the talkative extrovert.

Kent, a prominent American homeopath, wrote in the early 20th century, "Leave the patient in freedom always. Do not put any words into his mouth. Never allow yourself to hurry a patient; get into a fixed habit of examination, then it will stay with you. It is only when you sustain the sharpest kind of work that you can keep your reputation and fulfil your highest use. Say as little as you can, but keep the patient talking and keep him talking close to the line. If he will only talk, you can find out symptoms in general and particular. If he goes off, bring him back to the line quietly and without disturbing him."[10] This is the ideal towards which every homeopath strives.

Some of you might benefit from encouraging comments such as, "...and then...?" or more directly, "And what else?" or even, "Can you describe that again so that I can picture it more clearly?" Allow the story of your companion to arise undisturbed, unchanged by your own internal attitudes, or those of your homeopath. Your role is not to tell your homeopath what you *think* is the cause of your animal's illness. You are striving to depict the patient's image completely and without judgment.

You are there to tell your veterinarian what you see, hear, feel and smell.

Good homeopaths allow their minds to curl around the story of your animal companion. They leave themselves at the door and just follow the tempo of the story you are telling. This waiting, listening and observing allows the patient's story to emerge with clarity and exactness. No force required, no heavy-handed directing—the homeopath is simply being present and observing.

• • •

What next? I am ready to begin my study. I will use Hogarth's interview to generate a timeline and a symptom list, which will be central to managing his case for the rest of his life.

Timeline

The timeline lists the life history of the patient. It includes the dates of significant events such as birth dates, surgeries, treatments, vaccines, and most importantly, the first occurrence of each symptom. The timeline reveals whether a symptom recurred frequently or whether it was a one-time event that was rapidly suppressed. Past health records from other veterinarians are very helpful when filling in the timeline, as they enable your practitioner to discover long-forgotten first symptoms and the timing of historical events. The timeline brings to light the unique development of disease in your particular animal. From the quiet beginnings of minor seemingly unimportant indispositions such as runny noses and itchy ears, to more serious deeper affections of internal organs, and then ultimately to pathology, your veterinarian can see the patient's total story revealed.

Beyond a guide to the important landmarks in your animal's life, what is the advantage of a good timeline? This important document is a handy reference during treatment follow-ups, especially when symptoms arise that were not present at the intake. When a new symptom occurs, your homeopath will refer to their patient's timeline to determine when this symptom was last seen. During homeopathic treatment, the body will produce symptoms from the past that were not cured, and this presentation is typically in the reverse order of the symptom's recurrence. This means that more recent symptoms will come back first, followed over time by older and older symptoms. This is referred to as Hering's Law, and is based on observations of patients and how they respond to homeopathic treatment. This law is not immutable, because symptoms may come and go or even overlap, but it is a guide that comes in handy when evaluating the patient's response during treatment. This law reminds us that the body has a memory of its path to illness, and this is the same path over which healing will travel, in reverse.

• • •

Hogarth's timeline:

2005	birth year
2006	adopted; fear of loud noises; heavy shedding
8/10	moved to a new house
10/10	lethargy, whining, hindquarter lameness? treated with antibiotics
4/11	tiny mass on left ear flap
6/11	porcupine quills in nose
2/12	slowness to rise first seen here?
5/26/12	episode of laying on floor moaning; hard to get hindquarters up; treated with Rimadyl and antibiotics; began sneezing with greenish cloudy goo from the right nostril
6/28/12	profuse bleeding from the right nostril
9/15/12	dry nose began (externally)
10/12	now gurgling in throat and a hard lump discovered on bridge of nose
10/26/12	homeopathic intake interview

• • •

This timeline will be a handy guide throughout Hogarth's life. We see here that his excessive shedding isn't something new, but that it was evident before all of his other symptoms emerged. If Hogarth can be cured, his shedding will likely be the last symptom to clear up, because the body often heals in the reverse order that it got sick. Also, the remedy must cover this symptom to cure, since he's had it all his life. If he had just begun to shed as an adult, this symptom would not carry the same weight, because it could simply be due to his diet, rather than a signpost of early chronic disease present during his early life and continuing steadily to the present.

Now it's time to generate Hogarth's symptom list.

Symptom List

A symptom list is a judicious summary of the intake interview.

Now that I have my intake interview and my timeline, how can I keep this information at my fingertips? By creating the symptom list. This describes all the symptoms in detail which characterize the disease in the patient. It's your homeopath's chance to organize her voluminous intake interview notes and put them into a quick reference guide containing all the important points in the case. Each homeopath may organize her notes differently—one might organize by body system, others by the severity of the symptom, or from internal symptoms outward, but each symptom must be as completely characterized as possible. Any descriptive details are included alongside the pertinent symptom. Events which occur together (concomitants), such as Hogarth's snoring during the night, along with his bloody nasal discharge and sneezing, all are listed together to form a complete picture of the disease. This is your veterinarian's working template for determining the prescription. The symptom list must be unbiased, complete, and clear. It is the bedrock of the case. It is not a template for a particular remedy, but a unique description of this patient in his state of illness. This symptom list does not change over the years, except perhaps for more added symptoms if the patient gets sicker. This list contains the tracking points for follow-up consultations. Without this list, it is easy to get distracted by what's happening today, which can change from appointment to appointment.

The symptom list describes the patient from nose to tail and from top to bottom, including behavior and emotions.

Once your homeopath has the symptom list, they will keep it for the life of the patient. Kent wrote, "The physician who has in his casebook the notes of every illness of his patients, has wonderful hold of any community."[11] With a comprehensive and detailed symptom list, the patient's individual expression of disease is understood quickly and easily. A symptom list is never vague or ill-defined, because it is characteristic of the patient. "Vomiting and diarrhea" is an acceptable description in an allopathic clinic, but the homeopath may write, "Violent bouts of vomiting occurring in the early morning before eating breakfast, consisting of yellowish phlegm in small amounts and followed by listlessness. Diarrhea in the middle of the night accompanied by extreme restlessness, and, following the stool, great straining, for long periods." Specific, descriptive, vivid, and pointing right at the heart of the patient's disease. Here's an actual example from a patient: "[Stool] very watery, mucousy with a slight gelatin texture, paper bag brown, in chunks, sometimes with a horrific smell." Pretty dramatic! Each case of illness is unique to that individual, thus demanding a unique treatment.

The symptom list is not about diagnostic labels. Your homeopath will want to be well-informed about any diagnoses previously applied to your animal, but she will not need this information to determine the curative remedy. As Close writes, "The diagnosis of disease by modern methods is based largely upon physical signs, tests and reactions, involving the use of many instruments of precision, in which the patient takes no active part, and of which he has no knowledge. The selection of the homoeopathic remedy, on the other hand, is based very largely and sometimes almost entirely upon the phenomena [symptoms—what you see in front of you], or deductions drawn from the phenomena, of subjective, conscious experience, perceived only by the patient and stated by him to the examiner."[12] In other words, the results of blood work and radiographs (x-ray films) do not lead to knowledge of this particular patient's illness. A diagnosis does not help your homeopath determine the curative remedy. Treatment is based on what the patient demonstrates directly to you and to the homeopath.

Past Health Records—Necessary or Not?

Yes! From as far back in time as possible. As in any detective research, the more information the better. If your homeopath knows how your previous veterinarian has treated past illnesses, and which disease label has been used, she can direct her questions to you more specifically. So make that call to your traditional vet. These records are yours, so the request has to come from you, not from your homeopath. Health records enable your homeopath to see your animal over the years through the educated eyes of another professional. Interestingly, the notes left by veterinary technicians are often the most valuable, because they may list verbatim the description of the problem as told by you, years ago. Very helpful to the homeopath! These health records provide a year-by-year description of how chronic disease has developed in your animal, and also an indication of the route your animal may travel in her return to health.

It can be daunting to tell your allopathic veterinarian that you are planning to procure the services of a homeopathic colleague. But veterinarians are professionals. They understand that patients and clients may not stay with the same practice for years, and they are legally required to provide health records when requested. This request can often be handled painlessly by the front office staff, and nowadays it is often as simple as emailing electronic files. Your job is to provide all the information available about your animal to your homeopath, so that she has the best chance possible of selecting the proper remedy.

Past health records help fill in the blanks. Old forgotten illnesses, early symptoms occurring prior to the development of the presenting disease state (often found in "well" puppy and kitten visit records), timing of vaccines, dates of surgeries, all are important to determining the course of chronic disease in the patient. These records also document the frequency of office visits, which tells your homeopath how frequently the condition recurs, and how rapidly the patient is or is not declining. Finally, these records provide exact details of past treatments, which may have been forgotten in older animals. A patient having received multiple injections of a long-acting steroid will present differently and react differently to treatment than one who was not subjected to suppressive medicines.

To bolster the intake interview data, in addition to studying past health records, your vet might ask to talk to all available family members, breeders, or trainers. Even past guardians can often contribute, if they can be found and if they are willing. Their points of view can complement and sometimes illuminate yours.

• • •

What the homeopath needs to cure is the whole patient, in their unique state of suffering, with symptoms which may localize in more than one organ or body system. The symptoms, taken together to make up the whole, lead to the curative remedy. What stands out? What makes this cat or dog or horse or llama unique in her suffering? What has changed from her healthy days? How has she reacted to these changes? This is what characterizes the patient, and what must be found on her symptom list. A good symptom list, derived from the intake consult and past health records, is the touchstone that your veterinarian refers to during each follow-up. This list is close and personal, unique to your animal.

• • •

Hogarth's symptom list:

nasal discharge with sneezing
    green cloudy thick goo ("gucky"), then blood-tinged
    a gurgle in his throat
    blood (three times): first watery, then pure blood, "a cut"
    onset right side, now left also
    snores at night, when breathing out
    dry nasal sound, as if membranes swollen, when breathing in
    hard lump on bridge of nose
fears loud noises (guns, vacuum)
doesn't react on being pushed around by other dog (mellow)
hindquarters hard to get up in the morning on rising
    difficult to go downstairs (had to be carried in the past)
    laying down, moaning
smelly breath sometimes
heavy shedding
    dry coat
lies close to hot wood stove

• • •

Like a distillation, this list contains all the important tidbits from the interview, organized and ready for reference throughout the life of your companion. Notice that the symptoms are all observed directly through the senses of touch, sight, smell, and hearing. There are no interpretations, such as, "The other dog is the alpha, so he lets her push him around." Or, "She's always cold, so she snuggles against me the minute I sit down." Or, "She drinks from the faucet because she likes to play with the water." We don't know what our patients are thinking. We can guess, but it's only always a guess. What we see and observe is much more helpful, and leads more directly to the correct prescription. The more we guess about internal motivations and states of mind, the more shaky is our ability to match the patient with the treatment.

As astute observers, we can attribute basic emotions to our animals, such as fear, anxiety, rage, joy, and jealousy, but going further than that into the more complicated inner workings of their minds cannot be done with certainty. Even differentiating between anger and fear can be difficult, for example, in a an anxious dog who has learned to bite when provoked. For the purposes of homeopathic evaluation and treatment, stick to the facts and stay away from theories and guesses and assumptions.

• • •

Hogarth did benefit from homeopathic therapy, but he was not cured. The bleeding stopped and he continued to enjoy a good quality of life for another 16 months. At nine years of age, he was euthanized for a presumed cancerous growth in his nose. Right up until three days before he was euthanized, he was happy and vital and never left his beloved person's side.

• • •

Let's look at another interview, so that you can see how each one is different. This client, unlike the last one, is not new to homeopathic medicine. She readily fills in the blanks without my having to ask. This is Charlie, an 18 month-old intact male Bernese Mountain Dog, who came to me for itching and gulping.

Client: "This gulping is new. It's all of a sudden, with licking. Not the full attack like Berners get. It's at night after dinner, but it did stop a couple of days ago. He also has bright pink lips and skin, which is on and off. He's pink on his nose and belly. This I have seen before. His eyes get pink."

WJ: [Here I made a note to ask which came first, the itch or the pink skin, and where exactly "on his nose" means, since it would be very different if his nose leather was pink versus the skin around his nose.]

Client: "I think it's allergies."

WJ: [I don't interrupt here, even though this diagnostic information is not helpful, because I will interrupt the flow of her thoughts and perhaps cause a defensive reaction. Her focus is on her dog, not on me, and that's where I want it.]

Client: "He is also shaking his head, a huge amount. Probably from an itchy ear. He is easy-peasy, the easiest dog I've ever had. Even when he is pet, his back leg is scratching, but it's not constant. Today his itching is not too bad. His ears get pink, but there is not a lot of stuff in them. He rubs into his right ear and moans."

WJ: [See how naturally she gave me more details about how his ears feel, and how he reacts to the feeling? At this point I might ask at what age she first saw this itching and head shaking.]

Client: "He is really good at reading other dogs. Also he's sensitive to noise, for example wood cracking in the cold. He runs off the deck. If I open the door to let him in, he will fly into the house to get over the deck."

WJ: [Such a vivid portrayal of his reaction to noises! At this point she had stopped talking, so I asked for more details about how he reacts to other noises.]

Client: "He may startle if there is a loud bang, but not badly. He may run out of the kitchen, but then come back. He is fine with thunderstorms, fireworks, and guns."

WJ: [Again she seemed finished, so I prompted her by asking about what he was like as a pup.]

Client: "He hates, always, to have his feet touched. The Lyme disease settled there. With training it got better, but way worse with the Lyme again. He didn't like the car when I first got him. He screamed. He got over this quickly. He was so excited about Mannie [her other dog]. We kept them separated with gates, as he wanted to chew on Mannie's head. When they were ready to be together, they played."

WJ: [I referred to the pinkness on his nose that she had concerns about to get her talking again, asking when she first saw it.]

Client: "The pink on his nose (she refers to his upper lip next to his nose) has always been there. Bright pink. It did happen before this fall, maybe when he was hot? As a baby he fell in a hole and hurt himself. He cried! He is definitely sensitive to pain, which is normal."

WJ: [No need to argue, but I never take "normal" for granted. I just write down what is reported.]

Client: "When he had Lyme, he would cry to stand up, and cry if he moved a certain way. He will sit on my lap for a few minutes at night."

WJ: [At this point I make a note to ask more about his sensitivity to pain. I will want to know more details, how Charlie manifests it, and what helps him when he is in pain. But not until she is finished with her story.]

Client: "He prefers to be around me more than Mannie does. He stays with me outside or inside in the same room. He loves training. Once he was so distracted with the other dogs that he made high crying noises and wouldn't take a cookie, but now he is relaxed and unconcerned."

WJ: [Again she's stopping, so I ask about his appetite.]

Client: "Fantastic."

WJ: [I start into other areas of the body before zeroing in on particular areas of interest.] "What about any coughing and sneezing?"

Client: "No, but last night he did cough or hack for 15 – 20 seconds. He may hack treats back up. He doesn't chew. He gets them with clicker training, and it happens right after he is fed the treat."

WJ: "Tell me about other vomiting or diarrhea."

Client: "None."

WJ: "How is his sleep?"

Client: "He sleeps well. He drinks a lot, always has, at class and at home. He drinks for awhile, taking multiple drinks between 6 and 8pm. But on weekends I see him drinking all day." [At this point I make a note to ask where the client is during the day. If she works, then Charlie's drinking a lot between 6 – 8 pm is not as unusual. That's when she's home to see it.]

WJ: "What about his coat?"

Client: "Great. He doesn't like baths. Last time he actually cried. He tries to get away, and may not even take a treat."

WJ: [See how my questions bring out more information without more specific directions from me? She's already telling me when this behavior began ("always has") and giving me great details about what time of day things may happen.] "How is he with weather?"

Client: "For wind he's OK. There are no extremes in his behavior. He may not pant when Mannie did when it's 50 degrees in January."

At this point we are done with the natural flow of the story, so I continue with some more specific questions, such as what has been Charlie's experience with abdominal gassiness, and how about odors to his body, and tell me about his teeth and gums. Then, finally, the client has said all she came to say. I ask if there is anything more, just to be sure. If there is nothing more, then I go back over my notes to fill in as many details as I can. In Charlie's case, I want to know about his sensitivity to pain. So I asked her to describe this in more detail.

Client: "As a pup, when he was picked up a lot to see if he would yelp or not after getting chiropractic treatment, he would start running away if he thought you were going to pick him up again."

WJ: "What does he do when he's in pain, like after he fell in the hole?"

Client: "There are big sighs, and he leans on my shoulder while I'm holding him."

WJ: [Such a clear picture of the comfort he gets from being closely held! Much more quality information than if I had written, "Sensitive to pain."]

Client: "When he had the Lyme he was limping and screaming."

Then I wanted to know how he reacts to his feet being touched. Whenever I hear, "He likes...." or "She doesn't like...." I ask how the client knows this. I'm not challenging their knowledge, but simply gathering illustrative material so that I can judge the progression of the case in the future. It is much easier to know the details of the patient's reaction so that I can clearly measure improvements. Otherwise I can only ask whether the sensitivity has improved, and by how much. She answered, "He pulls his foot away, and then he may back away and move his body to get his foot out of my reach." Nice clear details, so clear that I can "see" it happening right in front of me, even though we are not touching Charlie!

My next question was about his screaming in the car as a pup.

WJ: "When during the ride did he scream?"

Client: "The last twenty minutes of the ride home. Then he vomited. He was OK by the fourth ride."

WJ: [I was glad I asked, because I had assumed that he screamed when he was first put in, but here we see that he began screaming only towards the end of the ride, and that this reaction involved vomiting. I also want to know his current state, for symptoms that have been coming and going, so that I will be able to determine what exactly changed at the follow-up, after the first prescription.]

Client: "Oh, sometimes he will be lying on the rug and jump up like something bit him, and act a little spooky. As a baby it took him twenty minutes to recover. Now it only takes one minute. I've seen this two times in the past six months."

As you can see, more information just floated up. I wouldn't have known to ask about this! As a client experienced in homeopathy, she knows to tell me the frequency of this behavior, and when it was first observed. Now we might be done! However, I always keep the door open by telling the client to contact me if they remember anything else.

• • •

Charlie's timeline:

7/18/11	birth date
9/11	brought home; screamed in car; no vaccinations; big drinker; sensitive to feet being touched; pink upper lips
9/17/11	fell in hole, screaming; ameliorated by being held
9/27/11	slipped on floor; screaming and crying
10/20/11	had a "cold"
10/26/11	distemper/parvo vaccine
2/1/12	rabies vaccine; then 2/5/12 acutely lame and temp of 104.0 F (normal is 101.8 F)
3/7/12	liquid diarrhea
5/12/12	mushy bowel movement; Lyme test positive; lameness
8/20/12	white around right eye got very red; upper lips especially bright pink
10/12/12	itch began and occasional sneezing and shaking; red right eye with discharge; panting
11/14/12	lame after falling spread-eagled
12/4/12	lethargic, lame in front limbs, temperature 104.0 F; administered antibiotics for presumed Lyme disease
1/13	gulping
2/1/13	homeopathic intake interview

• • •

What stands out in this timeline is how often this dog vocalizes when he is hurt. He is very dramatic. He has also had very little vaccines, which is unusual. Minimizing vaccines is a wise choice in any patient (we will discuss vaccines in the Supportive Care chapter), but especially important for Charlie, as he reacted with lameness and a fever a few days after his rabies vaccine. Good to know! Notice also that the reason he came to see me, his gulping, is only the latest (not the only) symptom in his short life.

• • •

Charlie's symptom list:

sensitive
  to pain
  to feet being touched
  cries if moves a certain way
  screams and limps easily, holding him helps
  runs past wood that had cracked in the cold (loud sound)
doesn't like baths
jumps up as if bit and acts spooky
creeps around other dogs sometimes, as if fearful
itchy
  panting
  red belly
  scabs after scratching
  shaking head a huge amount
  itching alternates with lameness in front limbs
  red eyes with clear goopy discharge
  fur loss around left eye
pink on upper lips
as pup, had a "cold"
  runny nose, some sneezing,
  goopy eye discharge, white goop under eyes on waking
diarrhea as pup

yelped as tried to defecate
mushy, liquid
concomitant: vomiting
drinks large amounts often, any time of day
gulping and licking after dinner
may hack up treats, then re-swallow them
lameness
holding up left front leg, lethargy, fever, suppressed with medications
umbilical hernia, large but can be pushed back in
screamed and vomited in car (as pup)

• • •

See how exactly each symptom is described? Also, symptoms which occur at the same time (concomitant symptoms) are listed together, showing the groupings. For example, when Charlie itches, this is often accompanied by panting and red eyes, and this itching often alternates with front limb lameness. Patterns of symptoms occurring together are very useful, as this furnishes more data points to match with the symptoms of the remedy.

Charlie has done well with homeopathic care, avoiding the lamenesses that seemed to trouble his puppyhood, and getting along much better with his housemate. He has had no further trouble with his skin, eyes, or ears, up to his current age of over three years old. There have been no further digestive issues or colds, though he still does remain sensitive to pain and to having his feet touched.

Why don't allopathic veterinarians ask all these questions? That's because the answers don't matter when you have been trained to use symptomatic therapy. Most veterinarians do not want to load their clients and patients up with expensive medications and their attendant side effects. So in my early years of allopathic practice, I might give Charlie a tranquilizer for his emotional sensitivity, or even a mood-altering drug, an anti-nausea drug for car rides, also an ointment for his ears. Definitely cortisone for his itching, maybe an antibiotic for his scabs, eye drops for the goopy discharge, and an antacid for gulping and licking after dinner. He might also need a pain killer or a nonsteriodal anti-inflammatory medication for his lameness.

That covers certain symptoms, but for other things allopathic medicine has no answer. What about the itching alternating with lameness? How about his fur loss that is only around his left eye? And his history—diarrhea and a runny nose—-these are past symptoms, so the allopath does not need to learn about those now. But the homeopath wants to know everything, because her treatment is selected based on current issues as well as past illnesses. The remedy matches the whole patient in time.

• • •

In the next chapter, we will look more closely at how the case material is analyzed. We'll study another case and go over the procedure followed by your homeopath in order to match the patient with the right remedy.

• • •

Chapter 4 References

1. Mosse K. Labyrinth. Penguin Group; New York, NY, 2005: 408.
2. Hahnemann S. *Organon of Medicine, Sixth Edition*. Künzli J, Naudé A, and Pendleton P, eds. Blaine, WA: Cooper Publishing;1982: 84.
3. Close S. *The Genius of Homoeopathy.* New Delhi, India: B. Jain Publishers;1997: 172.
4. *Ibid.* 2, p. 85.
5. *Ibid.*, p. 84.
6. *Ibid.* 3, p. 176.
7. *Ibid.* 2, p. 85.

8. *Ibid.*, p. 87.
9. *Ibid.*, p. 86.
10. Kent J. *Lectures on Homoeopathic Philosophy*. Berkeley, CA: Homeopathic Educational Services;1979: 160 - 161.
11. Gypser KH. *Kent's Minor Writings on Homoeopathy*. New Delhi, India: B. Jain Publishers;1988: 239.
12. *Ibid.* 3, p. 168.

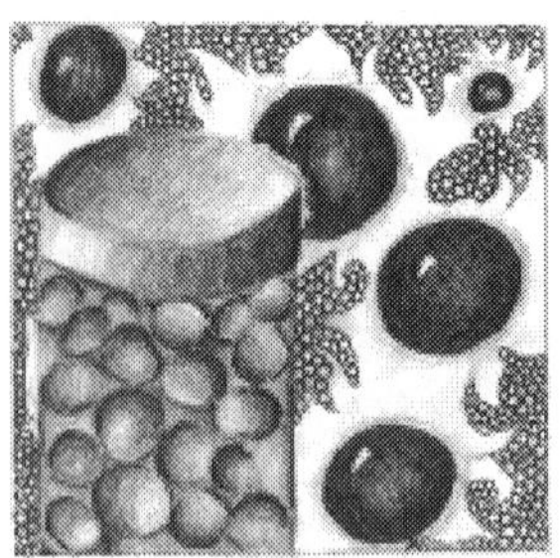

5 – Case Analysis

Case analysis enables a clear visualization of the patient's disease.

Now that the intake is complete, your homeopath will begin her study. She will separate wheat from chaff to gain a true image of the patient's disease. Not everything happening in the patient's body and mind directly points to the remedy which will heal him. For example, 177 remedies have watery diarrhea, but only one of these is the correct remedy for this particular patient. In addition, some idiosyncrasies of our patients are simply their normal personality traits which will continue into health. During case analysis, your homeopath will tease out the specific symptoms leading to the remedy. These are the characteristic symptoms.

The goal is to match the picture of your animal's illness, with *all* of its characteristic symptoms, to the curative remedy. An analogy might be identifying a certain group of skiers in a resort. You are comfortable in the lodge, with a good view of the slopes. You see a group coming down the hill that has the correct number of people. But that group isn't your family. Next you look for one skier in a group being much taller than the other two. Once you find that, you also look for the right colors, because one of your group wears a more unusual bright yellow coat. You might also notice that one is an expert skier and the others are slower and tend to turn more tightly back and forth across the steeper slopes. Do you see how the characteristics of the family group help you pick them out of a crowd of other skiing families? You don't look for people wearing helmets, because the majority of skiers wear them. You don't look for ski poles, for the same reason. You need to find the unusual, the unique combination, the identifying details that set your group apart. It is the same process when your homeopath is searching for a match between remedy and patient.

He will always look for the patient in the remedy, not the remedy in the patient, because he will find aspects of many different remedies in the patient. But what he needs to find is *all* the characteristic aspects of the patient in *one* remedy. In other words, he is not looking for all the family groupings that contain a yellow overcoat. He only wants the unique family grouping of three people, consisting of one tall person who is the expert skier, two who carve turns, and that bright yellow jacket.

Symptom List Analysis

The first step in case analysis is close study of the patient's symptom list. Symptoms guide us to the curative prescription. The symptom list in its entirety is used for patient follow-up, but only the characteristic symptoms are employed in the analysis. We monitor every symptom while treating the patient, but not every symptom guides to the remedy. How does your veterinarian know which symptoms are important? This chapter will discuss the difference between descriptive symptoms and prescription-guiding symptoms. Knowing what makes up a guiding, or characteristic, symptom will help you "see" your animal, and be better prepared to describe her symptoms to your homeopath.

What makes a symptom useful for understanding the case? Your homeopath is looking for those symptoms that are unusual, that stand out, or that have the most texture in tempo or quality or details. Characteristic symptoms are general ones pertaining to the whole body (also called generalities), followed by mental symptoms, and then peculiar symptoms. Less helpful are symptoms common to many diseases (like helmets and ski poles), and particular symptoms which pertain to one area of the body. We will discuss each of these in more detail below.

The Complete Symptom

A complete symptom tells us what it feels like, where it is, what makes it better or worse, and what other symptoms occur at the same time.

The complete symptom is often characteristic in a case. It has four aspects: location, or where in the body the symptom is expressed; modality, or what causes the symptom to be exaggerated or eased; concomitants, or other symptoms that occur at the same time as the main symptom under consideration; and finally the sensation associated with the symptom. This last aspect is often unavailable for use by veterinary practitioners, though we can get a sense of whether the pain, for example, is sudden or gradual, based on the behavior of the patient.

"A single symptom is more than a single fact; it is a fact, with its history, its origin, its location, its progress or direction, and its conditions."[1] This means you have to find out when the symptom began (its origin), how it changed over the life of the patient (its history), how it changed in response to previous treatments (its progress or direction), and what affects its expression (its conditions or modalities). Also be alert for other symptoms which go along with it. Your homeopath is selecting what is most important in your animal's story, or what most closely characterizes the patient's disease.

The Complete Symptom: Location

Where does the symptom originate? For example, some dogs only have warts on their chins, thus making the chin an important aspect of the case. Or perhaps the major complaint of a feline patient is in the nail beds. This location is then pertinent to the case. If a symptom is poorly described and yet clearly localized, the location itself can be useful to the practitioner, as will be shown later in the chapter.

Vomiting is localized in the stomach, and excess salivation in the mouth, and more complicated conditions such as diarrhea might be localized to the abdomen or the rectum. Where is the discomfort most acutely experienced by the patient? A dog experiencing prolonged straining after each movement has the disease located in the rectum, rather than the abdomen. Another dog may suffer from watery diarrhea which is preceded by loud rumbling in the abdomen, thus having the latter as the focus, or location, of his disease.

The Complete Symptom: Modalities

What eases you? Or what aggravates the symptoms? These are modalities.

Modalities are a difficult concept to master. They describe what makes the symptom better (amelioration) or worse (aggravation). Modalities also delineate the onset, inciting cause, or what brings on the symptom. These can have to do with the entire patient as well as a single symptom. Think about your own modalities. What time of day do you do your best work? Do you feel happiest when the whole family is home, or do you prefer solitude? Do you feel better when you are soothed, or do kind words simply make you grind your teeth? When you have pain, do you elevate the sore part, or cover it in warm blankets? After getting chilled, do you invariably come down with a chest cold? In medical school, we are not trained to look for what helps or aggravates a symptom, since this information has no relationship to allopathic medicine selection. But to match remedies, the modality is the icing on the cake. A clear modality, often characteristic to the patient, can be a valuable guide to the right remedy. They make the patient's picture stand out.

"By Modality we mean the circumstances of occurrence, aggravation and amelioration of any abnormal sensation reported by the patient [or in the case of veterinary practitioners, the client]. Amongst the modalities, causative factors, predisposing as well as precipitating, rank first; the aggravations come next, while the ameliorations are considered last. The modalities often furnish us with the much needed differentiating clues in a group otherwise considered as homogenous. Thus, from the standpoint of individualization, modalities assume the highest importance and a successful homoeopathic prescription will be determined by the ability of a homoeopathic physician to elicit and to evaluate them correctly. This is one of the most difficult tasks for a homoeopathic physician; very often, lack of observation, on the part of the patient or the physician leaves this vital data out of the picture."[2]

Modality descriptions often begin with the phrase, "He feels better (worse) when..." What affects your cat or dog's well-being? When is she most happy? What makes him afraid? Does eating a meal bring on her symptoms (diarrhea, vomiting, abdominal pain, etc.)? Does she become clingy when she's sick, or does she get snappy and irritable? These questions get you thinking about what aggravates or what ameliorates the disease.

A symptom can change according to the time of day, or sleeping versus waking, or even the weather or the season. The patient could be affected by the emotions of people around her, or the discipline involved with training. Some patients like to be coddled and soothed, others prefer being alone. Often modalities are similar across symptoms, which means they can be generalized to the whole patient. These are the most valuable modalities of all. For example, a dog may allow bathing of an infected eye with warm water, and also like warm applications on a hotspot. This same dog may love warm baths. This modality then becomes general, which holds more importance to the case than a modality applying to a single symptom. We will discuss generalities later in the chapter.

Hahnemann describes modalities in A. 133, "In order to define a particular medicinal symptom with precision, it is helpful and indeed necessary when experiencing it to place oneself in varying circumstances and to observe whether it increases, decreases, or disappears from movement of the affected part, from walking indoors or in the open, from standing, sitting, or lying; whether or not it tends to return when one reverts to the earlier circumstances; whether it is modified by such things as eating, drinking, speaking, coughing, sneezing, or other bodily activities; at what time of day or night it tends to be particularly evident. In this way the individual characteristics of a symptom become apparent."[3]

• • •

Examples of Modalities

cats who like to be touched only in the mornings, the rest of the day are fearful or easily irritated [ameliorated waking, ameliorated morning]

a cat who allows inexpert handling (as from a loving young child), yet fights tooth and nail against having blood drawn [aggravated from contradiction, aggravated from emotions (anxiety, fear, anger)]

dog who attacks, but only right after a seizure (read Sire's case later in this chapter) [worse after a seizure, worse when anxious]

dog who scratches frantically, but only when gently corrected [aggravated by anger, aggravated from emotions, aggravated from contradiction]

Practice looking for modalities in your animal. Notice when her stomach growls the loudest, or when he's hardest to train, or when she likes being carried around. Do these happen only when she is hungry? Find out if she eats better when the food is warm, or if he likes to lay quite close to the stove in the winter. Modalities are interesting and unique, bringing texture to your observations. Enjoy the detective work!

• • •

The Complete Symptom: Concomitants

Concomitants are symptoms that occur at the same time.

Concomitant symptoms occur together. For example, diarrhea and vomiting, or constipation and a lack of appetite, or shivering and anxiety. This is another way of describing a symptom more completely. "Concomitant symptoms are those that accompany the chief complaint but are not considered of much consequence by the patient as they do not bother him to the same extent. The only relationship that concomitants bear to the chief complaint is their occurrence at the same time."[4]

Examples of concomitants are found in the cases described in this book. For example, Charlie's itching (from the Intake Consultation chapter) has the following concomitants: panting, red eyes with a clear goopy discharge, red abdomen, scabs after scratching, and shaking his head a huge amount. Mandrake's dry barking cough (later in this chapter) is associated with a reduced appetite, chilliness, and front limb lameness. See how the concomitants are not part of the associated symptom? For example, an itchy ear with redness of the flap and swelling down in the ear canal are not concomitant symptoms, but rather, all part of the same symptom having to do with the ears. Itchy ears and lameness, however, are concomitants. Another example is Tiberius' emotional testiness with other cats, concomitant to his respiratory symptoms (later in this chapter). Concomitants are a valuable addition to the symptom list, and very helpful when searching for the curative remedy.

The Complete Symptom: Sensations

This is the final aspect of the complete symptom. Unfortunately, sensations are often unavailable to veterinary practitioners. The sensation is accessible only to those homeopaths who can communicate directly with their patients. "An abnormal sensation experienced by the patient in any particular part of the body or by the patient in general furnishes a clinician with the best evidence of disease. A homoeopathic physician is particularly interested in the abnormal sensations, which cannot be readily explained on the basis of the pathological changes that have occurred; they indicate to him the individuality of the patient on which the selection of the similar remedy rests. At times, the very intensity of a sensation marks it as a characteristic feature."[5]

Human patients might describe a buzzing, clenching, pricking, or pounding sensation, for example, perhaps associated with a headache or abdominal distress. In our animal patients, we can often see the *results* of sensations. The patient may point his nose suddenly to an area of concern, even nibbling the skin, which indicates that the sensation approaches rapidly and is somewhat intense. Animals also indicate sensation vocally, which is another hint to the astute client. But this aspect of the complete symptom is often either crudely ascertained, or entirely absent in the veterinary case.

General Symptoms

Generalities, or general symptoms, refer to "I" rather than "my."

General symptoms are very helpful to the homeopath, often serving as a reliable guide to the curative remedy. General symptoms involve the entire body, thus they might have to do with sleep, the sex drive, mental processes, emotions, or body temperature, such as chilliness or sweating (dogs and cats sweat on their foot pads, but this symptom can be generalized, unless only one foot is involved). In reference to human patients, "The General symptom is the one which is experienced by the patient as a whole; the patient does not refer to these complaints with 'my'; on the contrary, 'I' takes its place when the patient talks of these complaints. It will be apparent that the general symptoms will tend to depict the patient as a whole and hence will be of greater value in homoeopathic prescribing."[6] The client, referring to the patient, will also use pronouns when describing a general symptom, such as "he" or "she," rather than "his...(tail)" or "her...(paw)." Thus the statement, "She lays so close to the stove that her whiskers are singed," depicts a general symptom, whereas, "Her leg feels cold to the touch," is a particular symptom, which we will cover next.

• • •

Categories for General Symptoms

mental and emotional symptoms
intelligence
personality traits (when exaggerated)
sociability to animals and people
fears (of thunderstorms, noises, strangers, wind, touch, being looked at)
energy level
strength
gait and movement disorders
thirst
appetite
special cravings
body weight issues
reproductive issues
grooming habits (especially cats)
preference for heat or cold
sleep disturbances
growth and development

• • •

Mental and Emotional Symptoms

A type of general symptom, the mental and emotional symptoms, are also very useful to your homeopath. Memory, emotions, reactions during training, relationships, interactions with others, all involve the mind and the mental faculties. Mental symptoms can be difficult to distinguish from physical general symptoms in our animal patients. As observers, it is hard to differentiate when an animal is feeling better in her mind versus in her body. However, both are important states and the differentiation is not always critical. To ascertain mental and emotional states, your homeopath might ask about likes and dislikes, fears, what happens when the doorbell rings or when it's time to load onto the trailer, or how your animal reacts during training. The best way to answer these questions is to simply report what you see. Avoid interpretation whenever possible, for this is fraught with peril, and may lead to incorrect prescriptions. Report what you observe, not what you think your patient is thinking.

For example, you believe your dog is grieving the loss of a companion. Tell this to your homeopath, but then talk about why. What do you see in your animal that speaks of grief? Hiding, lack of appetite, irritability, sleeping more? Notice and report specific behaviors or expressions, rather than interpretations.

Peculiar Symptoms

Peculiar symptoms give you pause. You cannot explain them away.

Peculiar symptoms can also be very helpful to your homeopath. These are often characteristic of the right remedy. Peculiar symptoms stand out by their unusual nature, or their unexplained intensity. Examples from the cases in this book include the discharge of pure blood from Hogarth's nose, described as "a cut," which alternated with a mucousy discharge; Sire's furious violence after his seizure (especially considering his otherwise mild demeanor—see later in this chapter); Charlie's fur loss around only one eye (Intake Consultation chapter); Mandrake's tendency to bounce off walls in the clinic or off his guardian's back when he's hungry; and a cough during his lameness (see later in this chapter). Peculiar symptoms cannot be explained away, as could sweating during a fever, say, or anxiety when reprimanded. For this reason, peculiar symptoms are helpful indicators of remedies, because they delineate the nature of the patient's disease more clearly than common symptoms, which we will discuss next. They make the patient unique.

A. 153 reminds the practitioner that "...the more *striking, strange, unusual, peculiar* (characteristic) signs and symptoms in the case are especially, almost exclusively, the ones to which close attention should be given, because it is *these above all which must correspond to very similar symptoms in the symptom list of the medicine being sought* if it is to be the one most suitable for cure."[7]

A. 154 concludes, "If the corresponding image found in the symptom list of the nearest medicine contains in greatest number and most similarly the singular, uncommon, truly distinctive (characteristic) symptoms to be covered in the disease being treated, then *this* medicine is the most suitable one, the specific homoeopathic remedy for *this* case, and one dose of it will usually remove and extinguish a fairly recent disease, with no significant ill effects."[8] Unfortunately, most of our veterinary cases are inherited disease, thus requiring more than one dose of remedy, but the benefits of relying upon strange, rare, and peculiar symptoms still apply. Kent writes, "The things that characterize are things to make you hesitate, to make you meditate."[9]

Common Symptoms: Less Helpful to the Case

Common symptoms, on the other hand, do not guide to the proper remedy. These symptoms are easily explainable and not peculiar to the patient, such as weight loss in feline hyperthyroidism, or frequent urination during bladder inflammation. Common symptoms typically have no clear modalities, thus making them much less useful in the case. For example, a cat with kidney disease who is drinking a lot will not be unusual, because cats with compromised kidneys almost always show increased thirst. This symptom is very common, thus a less important guide to treatment. As another example, a racing heart is not useful as a guiding symptom in a hyperthyroid cat (this is a very common symptom in this condition), just as a saggy abdomen need not get your attention in a dog with adrenal problems, because these patients typically have low abdominal muscle tone. Whereas a thirsty cat with healthy kidneys is much more peculiar, since cats typically don't often head to the water bowl unless they are fed only dry food. Unusual and unexplainable symptoms are more useful in determining the curative remedy.

Your veterinarian will still follow up on these common symptoms, asking you how they are progressing, to help determine the patient's progress. However, they do not serve as a guide to treatment. Keep in mind that a common symptom can masquerade as a peculiar symptom, until it is seen in context. Here Kent describes how easy it is to label a symptom peculiar if the interview stops before the final question is answered, "In sicknesses the symptoms that cannot be explained are often very peculiar; the things that can be accounted for are not so often peculiar; peculiar things are less known to man. For instance, a patient can sit only with his feet up on the desk, or with his feet elevated; he is a great sufferer, and because of this suffering he is compelled to put his feet up. The symptoms hence will be put down, worse from letting the feet hang down. 'Well, what do you mean by that? Why, if I let my feet hang down, I find I bring the nates [buttocks] down upon the chair, and there is a sore place there.' Now that is quite a different thing. You many find if it is an old man that he has a large prostate gland, which is very painful at times and very sore, and when he lets the feet hang down the gland comes in contact with the chair. So we see that the real summing up of the case is that this enlarged and sore prostate gland is worse from pressure, and all you have learned from that symptom is that the gland is sensitive to touch, which is a common symptom. There are instances, however, where by letting the feet hang down the patient is ameliorated; for instance, you take a periostitis [pain in the bone] and the pain is relieved by letting the limbs hang. No one can tell why that limb is better when hanging over the bed. He lies across the bed with the foot hanging over the side, and why it is that he cannot lie upon his back nobody can figure out."[10] Thus, this symptom is peculiar, not common.

Particular Symptoms: Also Less Helpful to the Case

Particular symptoms are those affecting a part of the body, rather than the patient in his entirety. Ear inflammation, or a corneal condition, or gingivitis are all particular symptoms. When taken alone, particular symptoms are not as helpful as general symptoms with modalities, but when a group of particulars all share a similar quality, then this can be generalized, making the job of the practitioner much easier. For example, a patient with a greenish eye discharge who also has a green vaginal discharge and a purulent nasal discharge, must have green discharges in her remedy. As Kent puts it, "...after you have gathered the particulars of every region of the body, and you see there are certain symptoms running through the particulars, those symptoms that run through the particulars have become generals, as well as particulars. Things that apply to all the organs may be predicated of the person himself. Things that modify all parts of the organism are those that relate to the general state."[11] So particulars, in and of themselves, may not be useful, but if they make a pattern when grouped together with other particulars, then they become quite valuable.

As another example, Kent writes, "The patient says, 'I have so much burning,' and if you examine him, you find that his head burns, that the skin burns, that there is burning in the anus, burning in the urine, and whatever region is affected burns. You find the word burning is a general feature that modifies all his sickness. If it were only in one organ, it would be a particular, but these things that relate to the whole of the man are things in general."[12] The "things in general" are general symptoms, which are valuable indeed.

• • •

Let's look a a case example of a complete symptom, which is a fully-described alteration in the state of our patient's health. To review, complete symptoms consist of location, modalities, concomitants, and sensations (the latter often absent in veterinary cases). Here is an example, in a young dog with chronic diarrhea:

• • •

Harriet's symptom list:

location: gastrointestinal system
modality: worse in the middle of the night

concomitants: "awful" accidents, "a dribble here, a dribble there;" wakes up panting and whining

particulars: stool is very watery, mucousy with a slight gelatin texture, "paper bag brown," in chunks, and sometimes with a "horrific" smell

• • •

Harriet is an example of a case with particulars that are peculiar, and thus useful to the case. Harriet is truly incontinent with this diarrhea, as shown by her accidents and dribbling. She is obviously upset by the condition, showing this by panting and whining. The curative remedy must have a focus on the intestinal tract, along with incontinence and mental distress.

Harriet's diarrhea resolved after one dose of her remedy.

• • •

We've discussed the types of information most valuable to your homeopath. After collecting the characteristic symptoms, what happens next? Repertorization, or matching the characteristic symptoms in the patient with the characteristic symptoms of the remedy. This will be discussed in the following chapter, Repertorization.

Now that you see how carefully the symptoms are studied in the case, let's examine another intake. Here are the main points of the interview, before I had asked any questions:

• • •

Sire, a three year-old neutered male German Shepherd dog with seizures followed by aggression:

obtained from a reputable breeder at 13 months of age

present body weight of 91 lb., which is a good weight for him

this client is his fourth guardian

all previous guardians have been deployed military

one had a second dog
has jealousy issues, so client won't get another dog
first seizure was 4/22/10
grand mal (involving the whole body), lasting less than one minute
second seizure 5/2/10
really stiff, fell over, huffing and puffing as if he had run a mile
once tried to attack the client afterwards

• • •

The story has come to a pause. Look over this list and think about where you might want to fill in the blanks. I asked about how Sire had gotten along with his previous canine housemate, then I wanted to know more about his jealousy issues.

WJ: "How does he show jealousy?"
Client: "He'd go over to get attention if the other dog was getting it."
WJ: "What do you mean by 'attack'?" (this happened after the seizure)
Client: "He lunged at me, snapping, more scared, ran into the back of the house, confusion, not sure of what was going on."
WJ: "What happened after the second seizure?"
Client: "Took five minutes to come out of it, I'd move, he'd flinch, he'd move, I'd flinch, then he came out of it."

The picture becomes clearer as I draw out more details. I get to fully understand the degree of his jealousy as well as the situations that bring it out. As for the aggression after his seizure, we now have a clear idea of its severity, based on how careful and reactive the client was after the second seizure. I fill in the blanks with the client, not with my own imagination or previous experiences. It's easy to make Sire's jealousy or seizures just like the last cases of jealousy or seizures I have seen, because at vet school I was trained to look for the pattern, the common thread between patients. But homeopathic prescribing demands the knowledge of *individuality* in order to determine the curative treatment. That's where you come in, the person who lives with the patient, who shares walks and pets and lap time and socializing and training. You are the expert.

• • •

The final step in the intake is direct observation of the patient himself, including the physical examination. Dr. Close describes the details available to the astute clinician, or the informed client, writing, "If the patient is confined to bed [or unable to rise], the examiner will observe his position in bed, his manner of moving or turning, his respiration, the state of his skin, color or odor of perspiration [check the feet of dogs or cats], odor of exhalations from mouth or body, physical appearance of excretions, relation of the patient's sensations to atmosphere and temperature is shown in amount of covering, ventilation of room, ice bags, hot water bottle, etc., [you might find out whether these types of interventions help your animal]—all these, and many other little points, noticeable by the alert examiner, perhaps without asking a question, will be valuable guides in the choice of the remedy."[13]

• • •

Sire's timeline:

2007	year of birth
2008	adopted (had three previous homes); "life of the party," "jealousy issues"
2009	moved from one state to another
9/09	moved to present house
1/10	client had period of very stressful employment
4/22/10	first seizure, another one 5/2
5/7/10	homeopathic intake interview

• • •

This timeline is not as helpful as the ones from previous cases, since this dog's early records were unrecoverable. We do see, however, that the first seizure occurred shortly after the client had been severely stressed. Worth noting. Sire is an anxious dog (refer to his symptom list in the following pages). He can be skittish around thunderstorms and other loud noises, and he loves to be around people and other dogs. He lays close to the client when at home, and barks excitedly, pulling to get to other dogs when out on the leash. So he would definitely have been affected by the client's stress. He is an anxious reactive dog who likes company. This does not mean that anxiety causes seizures, but anxiety certainly could have caused Sire's chronic disease to become worse. Thus one of his modalities is "worse for anxiety." Also of interest is that he has changed homes often during his short life. More stressors that potentially have accelerated the development of his chronic disease.

As discussed before, the timeline is very helpful when seemingly new symptoms occur during treatment. If your veterinarian finds the "new" symptom in the timeline, he will be reassured that all is going well. (Remember how old symptoms return during a positive response to a remedy?) If the symptom is truly new, and persistent, then it may be one hint that the remedy needs changing. We will discuss more about what happens after a remedy administration in later chapters.

Hering's Law, introduced in the chapter Intake Consultation under "Timelines," reminds us that symptoms often resolve in the reverse order from which they appeared. The meticulously-crafted timeline graphically illustrates the appearance and disappearance of each symptom, providing your veterinarian with a clear guide to evaluate the progress of your animal's case. If symptoms are returning and then going away in the reverse order from which they first appeared, all is well. The timeline is your homeopath's guide. If, however, the patient seems to be responding well to the initial prescription, and then a very old symptom returns along with significant discomfort, this may cause your veterinarian much more concern than if the first returning symptom was a more recent one. The timeline grounds us in the story of your companion, providing hints to the unique path that he will take towards healing.

• • •

Sire's symptom list:

loves people, "hit of the party"
very vocal when excited, barks "not in play"
    pulls to other dogs when on a leash
anxious or fearful
    during loud noises or thunderstorms
    when something suddenly drops
    "really skittish," goes into his crate or paces
"abandonment issues" (old symptom)
    after boarding at a kennel, climbs into client's lap
    tries to climb out of car if left alone
seizures, followed by aggression
    fear after the seizures? (unsure)
    before seizures, restlessness
    "always touching me" (the client), but keeps moving his body
likes cold water, toilet water, running tub water (before it warms up)
prefers the cooler basement during hot weather
    sleeps in the shower stall at night
itching, skin flaky (This happened later on in the case after the first prescription, so I added it to the symptom list.)

• • •

Symptom lists are not perfect. Vets rely on you and the patient's health records to recall and accurately describe all the symptoms. Sometimes we have to make do with "abandonment issues," for example. This description might be accurate or it might not, but it reminds me to ask about how Sire does when left alone at future follow-ups. Working to help animals who do not speak our language is not an easy task. We all have a tendency to interpret our animal's symptoms, and often the interpretation takes on a life of its own. But the more we can stick to what we see, hear, smell, and feel, the more the symptom list will lead to the right remedy.

• • •

Notice the complete symptom in Sire's list (seizures), which is very helpful:

location: neurologic system
modality: during the night
concomitants:
  before seizure: restless, lays touching her, but keeps moving
  during seizure: really stiff, falls over, huffing and puffing as if ran a mile, bladder and bowels released
  after seizure: fear? tried to attack client when she approached him holding a towel; lunging and snapping, confusion, "[He is] not sure of what is going on," took five minutes to come out of it (these are mental symptoms as well as peculiar symptoms)

• • •

Sire is suffering from seizures, a general symptom, but the seizure itself is not characteristic. With most seizures, the patient becomes really stiff, falls over, and huffs and puffs. He may also experience involuntary urination and defecation. Often patients will be restless before the seizure, making this a common symptom and thus not so helpful for characterizing Sire's disease. What is peculiar is his history of extreme aggression after the seizure. Sire is a friendly dog and this behavior really stands out as unusual, not only for his personality when he is well, but for any post-seizure patient. Now we have a detailed and specific picture of this patient, rather than a one-size-fits-all seizure patient. This is critical before we go on to select the curative remedy.

• • •

In Sire's case, the closest match was the remedy sulfur. (We will discuss selection of the remedy in detail in the next chapter, Repertorization.) Here are the descriptions of sulfur in the materia medica which show how closely this remedy aligns to Sire's state:

sulfur:

Nerves: Uneasiness and excitation of nervous system; could not sit long; even while lying was constantly moving feet....convulsions after suppressed eruptions; often removes tendency to convulsions....[14] (These seizures recurred after Sire's skin condition disappeared, which is another hint supporting sulfur.)

Mind: Furiously mad; wanders about streets; after suppression of tinea capitis [an itchy scaly condition of the scalp] [15] Very much excited and very passionate.[16]

Appetite: Great thirst for ice cold drinks.[17]

Temperature: Cannot remain long in heated place....[18]

• • •

Sulfur was not Sire's first remedy, but it was the remedy that helped him the most. After a different prescription early on in his case, Sire began itching and his skin was flaking. We waited. When that condition stopped manifesting, his seizures returned. These skin issues, and their relationship to Sire's seizures, helped me fill out his case, making it possible to find his curative remedy. Suppression of a skin condition (Sire's itching and flaky skin) followed by aggravated symptoms (his seizures) is a hallmark of sulfur. The uneasiness described in sulfur also fits Sire exactly. In the client's words, Sire "lays touching me but keeps moving." This is extremely close to "even while lying was constantly moving feet...." Sulfur is a satisfying fit. In addition, this remedy is well known for being a thirsty remedy which desires cold water. Interestingly, there is a mention of being "furiously mad," though not in relation to the seizures. I would have preferred a more direct link between his emotional state and his seizures, but this is the remedy that matched his case, as shown by his positive response.

Sire, now eight years old, has done very well with sulfur. Once he was given this remedy, he had only one more seizure (the very next morning). He has been seizure-free for four years at the time of this writing, and has not needed another dose for the past 17 months.

• • •

Here is the case of Mandrake, a five year-old domestic shorthair cat who suddenly became unable to urinate. Examine his symptom list to see if he "comes alive" for you. The client is quoted directly when her description is particularly vivid.

• • •

Mandrake's symptom list:

- aggression
  - doesn't like to be confined
  - "bouncing off the walls in the clinic"
  - bounces off client's back when she is sitting on floor, "wreaking havoc"
  - might bite and claw if you want to get him off a chair
  - "a wild man"
- eats excessively
  - may put teeth on client's leg when waiting for dinner
- barking dry cough (local vet diagnosed bacterial pneumonia)
  - "rack" sound (to his cough)
  - onset after weather cooling off
  - concomitants (symptoms occurring at the same time as the cough)
    - pants after hard play
    - no longer playing; "energy slightly low"
    - appetite slightly less; "hasn't gobbled every bit lately"
    - chilly, laying on computer monitor and under light bulbs
    - limping on alternate front feet, walking "deliberately" as if painful

line of red on gums around upper right canine, dusky pink
dirty wax buildup in both ears
    itchy ears "holds one out sideways, stops and scratches"
abscess with bad smelling bloody yellow thick discharge (historical)
onset of illness (urinary difficulties) after exposure to cold and wet all night
    previously, tail slammed in truck door
    straining a long time, small amounts of urine
    urine dribbling out of him in car on way to hospital
    when struggling at vet's suddenly "ton of urine poured [out]"
    can express bladder manually but not fully emptying his own bladder
    concomitant: vomiting brown fluid

• • •

This list covers all the known areas in which Mandrake has expressed his illness, now and in the past. Not just symptoms involving his urinary system, but his respiratory system, his ears, and how he handles his emotions. Note also the detailed description of the discharge from his previous abscess. Types of discharges are very important in defining the disease state. Mandrake is a feisty cat with a large personality who doesn't do anything in a small way! See also the complete symptom in Mandrake's list, which will really help narrow the field:

• • •

Mandrake's complete symptom:

straining a long time to urinate, producing small amounts of urine
location: urinary bladder
modalities: onset following suppression of cough; also tail slammed in door; then exposure to cold and wet all night (Aggravated after suppression, possibly aggravated after injury; also aggravated by cold and wet

weather.)
concomitant: vomiting brown fluid

• • •

Mandrake presents like thousands of other cats with feline lower urinary tract disease, but what holds him apart and makes him unique is that with external help, he can urinate easily. This is a peculiar symptom. He is straining to urinate because his bladder isn't working right, rather than straining due to a blocked or constricted urethra. He was treated at the emergency hospital (the client was not local) with catheterization, but this did not resolve the problem, because he was suffering from bladder paralysis. The location of his disease was in the bladder, and the onset was after exposure to cold wet weather. So Mandrake's modality is bladder paralysis aggravated by exposure to cold and damp. Having a nice clear concomitant symptom in another location (his vomiting) is also very helpful to characterize Mandrake's case.

Notice that I did not characterize Mandrake as urinary incontinent, even though urine did pour out when he was struggling. When a patient with a very full bladder moves vigorously, it is normal for the bladder to release its contents. Dribbling in the car is another example: Mandrake (similar to most cats) was likely very stressed by riding in the car, and his overly full bladder would naturally leak as he moved about. If Mandrake was incontinent, he would have been dribbling urine right from the beginning, as he moved about his own house. So his urethra was doing its job and holding in the urine, until finally his bladder got so big that something had to give.

• • •

Now let's go back and look at his history to see how his illness manifested itself over time:

Mandrake's timeline:

9/04	jumped in the truck at a gas station; about eight months old; neutered shortly afterwards
10/04	drop in appetite, coughing, chill
5/06	abscess
12/12/06	tail slammed in truck door
1/3/07	caught out in cold and damp all night; straining to urinate; brought to emergency practice

• • •

See how all of Mandrake's past illnesses are included in his timeline, so that you can see the progression of chronic disease from a cough and skin infections to a condition which could have been fatal? The right remedy covers all of these conditions. Since male cats with urinary symptoms often look much the same on presentation, having detailed background information and descriptions of how this particular patient reacted to his illness is critical to selecting the best possible treatment.

• • •

Putting all of Mandrake's symptoms together, the closest remedy match was phosphorus. Here's the description of symptoms which read very close to his case:

Mandrake's materia medica:

phosphorus:
Urinary Organs: Bladder is full but urine does not flow because of absence of urging....[19]

Temperature: From warm to cold air: cough worse. Change of temperature...cough worse.[20]

Skin: Furunculosis [abscesses]; tendency to formation of boils; prevents formation of styes [red painful lump at the edge of the eyelid]; small purulent collections around ulcer; ulcer after boils on other parts of body.[21] (These all show the remedy's tendency to form infections and abscesses.)

Tissues: Lymphatic abscesses, full of fistulae [drainage sites at the skin]...pus copious and yellow.[22]

Hearing and Ears: A painful and inflamed gathering in right ear, first in left; matter and blood are discharged....[23]

Respiration: Breathing: very much oppressed, short; impeded by rapid walking; very short after coughing; tight after slightest food; short with violent pressive pain in upper part of sternum; difficult; superficial; anxious, panting, oppressed; anxious, short and hurried, with elevation of whole thorax, and especially of left side; very labored, noisy, panting.[24]

• • •

So what happened to the cat who picked out his new family from the line-up at a gas station? It was not a smooth transition to homeopathy. He had been in the veterinary hospital, getting catheterized and medicated with specifics. (Specifics refer to medicines given to address a single problem, such as urethral relaxants, anti-inflammatories, and antibiotics.) Mandrake had shut down. His bladder no longer reacted to the presence of urine, and he even stopped trying to urinate at all. When his bladder was pressed, urine dribbled out passively.

I gave him a single dose of 30C phosphorus, with excellent results, in spite of all his previous interventions. His bladder began working, he stopped scratching and biting, his lingering cough finally went away, and best of all for household serenity, he stopped using crouching people as launching pads before dinner. He needed no other remedy for another 2 ½ years.

• • •

Veterinary homeopathy, used correctly, can help with very serious conditions, as in Mandrake's case. This next cat had something filling up his chest. Without needing to spend thousands of dollars on diagnostics, I was able to help this cat, guided only by his symptoms. Meet Tiberius, a two year-old domestic shorthair cat, with a cough and a possible growth in his chest:

• • •

Tiberius' timeline:

2008	birth year
9/09	arrived at client's house; then neutered; had a scratchy voice
6/12/10	began coughing and sneezing, then his cold symptoms abated after steroids and antibiotics
7/12/10	began wheezing
7/28/10	intake consultation

• • •

Dates when certain symptoms were first seen are very useful to the homeopath. In Tiberius' case, his respiratory troubles began with a seemingly minor cold. Then the cold went deeper, from a sneeze to a lung wheeze. This progression is an important aspect to Tiberius' case, because the right remedy will only be found among those which describe respiratory issues that descend from the nasal passages into the lungs.

• • •

Tiberius' symptom list:

calm and unflappable
likes to snuggle in bed but then gets overheated and goes off on his own
drools when pet
scratchy voice
onset of illness: a cold; coughing and sneezing; then this went away
then began wheezing, with rattles "can hear it across the room"
right eye held somewhat closed and third lid raised
swallows extra, repeatedly, one minute after eating
since ill he's more testy with other cats; gets into fights
radiographs (x-rays) revealed a narrowed trachea
chest is non-compressible (a normal cat's chest can be gently compressed with little resistance—but do not try this without training)

• • •

Notice that Tiberius has a complete symptom in his list:

location: lungs
modality: disease began as a "cold" (coughing and sneezing), then this went away before wheezing began (wheezing following suppressed upper respiratory symptoms)
concomitants: right eye, held slightly closed with third lid showing (Horner's syndrome—see below); swallows extra and repeatedly one minute after eating; more testy (a mental symptom) with other cats; getting into fights (which is new)
peculiar: breathing rattles "can hear it across the room"

• • •

Tiberius shows a very specific order to the progression of his disease. His timeline, beginning with a cold and ending with a serious respiratory condition, characterizes his illness. Even before radiographs confirmed that his trachea was not in its normal position (suggesting that it was shifted by something in his chest), his physical exam findings made it clear that something serious was going on. Normal cats have a readily compressible chest, with flexible ribs that can be gently pressed in until the examiner can feel the heart beating (in experienced hands, this is not uncomfortable to the cat). Tiberius' chest would not compress normally. Also his Horner's syndrome indicated that the nerves to his eyelids were pinched (these come from the spinal cord and travel through the chest), thus causing his right eyelid to droop and his third lid to elevate. Luckily, Tiberius had concomitant symptoms to round out his case, namely a changed personality and repeated swallowing after eating. Whenever the personality changes during an illness, consider this a strong characteristic symptom that will be very helpful in your veterinarian's search for the healing remedy.

• • •

Notice that the categories under discussion merge and meld together. Concomitants, specifically, can also be peculiar symptoms in their own right, or general symptoms, or even mental symptoms. A mental symptom, such as Tiberius' increased testiness to others during his respiratory ailment, can also be interpreted as a modality: aggravated by company. It all depends on the focus of the case. Is Tiberius' illness in the mental plane or does it center around his lungs? What about Sire? Is his aggression part of his illness, or is he simply reacting to a frightening event? With experience, the practitioner learns to visualize the center of the case. The more refined this ability, the quicker the curative remedy will be found. This increased speed takes much study and many years of practice to develop.

Sulfur was the closest match to Tiberius. Here is what the materia medica describes for symptoms in the respiratory tract:

• • •

sulfur:

Respiration: Labored, heavy breathing....Rattling in chest....[25]

Throat: Dryness of throat: exciting cough; at night; constant desire to swallow saliva in order to moisten affected parts.[26]

Hahnemann: A dryness in the mouth and a scraping in the throat, as if the food would not go down....Accumulation of water in the mouth (sour and bitter).[27] Tightness of the chest.[28]

Kent: Many complaints come on from becoming warm in bed....[29] This remedy is full of difficult breathing, shortness of breath from very little exertion, copious sweat, so exhausted; asthmatic breathing and much rattling in the chest. Every time he gets "cold," it settles in the chest or in the nose....Every cold he takes ends in asthma.... [30]

• • •

Does this sound like Tiberius? A cat with a rattly chest who gets hot when snuggling too much at night, and swallows repeatedly after eating? Yes. A single 30C dose of sulfur transformed him from "working hard to breathe," to "seems fine to me," in two weeks. His eye came back to normal, he stopped fighting, and he began playing again. A few months later I checked his chest, and it was compressible, like that of a normal cat. He has not needed any other treatment in the past five years.

• • •

One hallmark of chronic disease is that it keeps coming back, without treatment aimed directly at the energetic level of the vital force. Various medications given to address the most bothersome symptom seem to help temporarily, but then the symptom recurs, worse each time. Homeopathy gets our animals off this merry-go-'round of symptomatic treatment.

• • •

In Kevin's case, he was a thirteen year-old cat with a chronic ulcer on his cornea. His caretaker had been fighting this condition for months without success. Eye ointments could not keep the ulcer away for long.

Kevin's symptom list:

right eye, non-healing ulcer

mild redness and swelling of the conjunctiva
squinting
tartar, gingivitis
hungry often, and overweight
hindquarter weakness, worse on the left side
exercises from the middle up
clumsy
uses his bulk to bully other cats
howls in travel carrier

• • •

Note that Kevin's appetite is discussed, along with his body weight. Just having some extra weight is not necessarily from chronic disease, but may only be from a poor diet and the lack of opportunity to exercise. But an adult cat who is often hungry, even though receiving enough calories to gain weight, may have an appetite problem as part of his illness. Something is out of balance.

• • •

Kevin's timeline:

2/28/97	birth date
8/97	declawed and neutered
8/05	anesthesia reaction during dentistry for tartar and gingivitis
8/08	lost 2 lb of body weight, hindquarter weakness
2009	first began to meow (some time during this year, unsure exactly when)
9/09	left ear flap swollen with blood (hematoma)
1/19/10	ulcer in right eye which never fully clears up
4/10	corneal edema (fluid buildup in the cornea that appears as an opaque whiteness)

5/10	began homeopathic treatment

• • •

Kevin's timeline and his symptom list tell us all we need to know to help him. Encompassing the mind, the emotions, and the physical planes, the body expresses the illness that saturates all of its levels, from energetic imbalances to functional disorders to pathology. The body as a whole is sick, and the symptoms are the language of this disease. If your veterinarian can clearly see the sickness, then he has taken the first and most important step towards finding the treatment. Your observations are critical to your homeopath's understanding. No-one else can give him the deep knowledge required in order to make the best possible match between patient and healing remedy. The knowledge is in you!

• • •

The remedy fitting Kevin's symptoms is calcarea carbonica, derived from the shell of the oyster.

Kevin's materia medica:

calcarea carbonica:
Sight and Eyes: Vascular ulcer on cornea. Ulceration of cornea in child with...distended abdomen.[31]
Constitution: Young who grow too fat and heavy.[32]
Kent: Muscles flabby....The Calcarea patient can't go upstairs; he is so tired in his legs, and so tired in the chest; he pants and suffocates from going upstairs. He has every evidence of muscular weakness and flabbiness.[33] Calcarea is a great friend to the oculist [person who treats eye conditions].[34]

• • •

Calcarea fits Kevin in multiple areas. It fits an overweight patient, but not just the weight—it fits the limitations imposed with his weight. Not being able to go upstairs, being tired in the legs, and panting and suffocating when he does go upstairs--this is an overweight patient who does not like to exert himself. This is exactly what Kevin looks like. Interesting that along with this more general symptom match is the mention of a corneal ulcer in this remedy.

Kevin had been struggling with his ocular ulcer for four months. His disease was not limited to his eye, however, as shown by his tartar and gingivitis, hind limb weakness, and an ear hematoma in his history. Calcarea covered all of these symptoms. After a single dose of 30C, he needed no further treatment for the next year and eight months, at which time a dose of 200C kept him well for another six months, until he was lost to follow-up. Kevin's ocular ulcer healed and never returned. But best of all, he became well in many other areas. He would stand up on his hind legs for attention, which was a big change from only exercising from the middle up! Also, he was able to jump two feet onto the arm of the sofa. He would come bounding down the stairs in the morning, and he was less aggressive to the other cats. He even lost a bit of weight as his appetite moderated. The clients described him as now preferring to look out the screen door instead of into the fridge. The right remedy heals the whole cat. No need for a lifetime of medication.

• • •

Chapter 5 References

1. Close S. *The Genius of Homoeopathy.* New Delhi, India: B. Jain Publishers;1997: 152.
2. Dhawale LD. *Principles & Practice of Homoeopathy.* Bombay, India: S.Y. Chougule; 1994: 66.
3. Hahnemann S. *Organon of Medicine, Sixth Edition*. Künzli J, Naudé A, and Pendleton P, eds. Blaine, WA: Cooper Publishing;1982: 113.
4. *Ibid.* 2, p. 60.
5. *Ibid.*, p. 64-65.

6. *Ibid.*, p. 61.
7. *Ibid.* 3, p. 125.
8. *Ibid.*, p. 126.
9. Kent J. *Lectures on Homeopathic Philosophy*. Berkeley, CA: North Atlantic Books; 1979: 204.
10. *Ibid.*, p. 206.
11. *Ibid.*, p. 209.
12. *Ibid.*, p. 207.
13. *Ibid.* 1, p. 181.
14. Hering C. *The Guiding Symptoms of Our Materia Medica*. Vol. 10. Paharganj, New Delhi, India: B. Jain Publishers;1995: 159.
15. *Ibid.*, p. 101.
16. *Ibid.*, p. 103.
17. Morrison R. *Desktop Guide to Keynotes and Confirmatory Symptoms* from *ReferenceWorks Pro*. [computer program] Version 4.2.5.2. San Rafael, CA: Kent Homeopathic Associates.
18. *Ibid.* 14, p. 164.
19. *Ibid.* 14 (Vol. 8), p. 352.
20. *Ibid.*, p. 381.
21. *Ibid.*, p. 395.
22. *Ibid.*, p. 393.
23. *Ibid.*, p. 339.
24. *Ibid.*, p. 359.
25. *Ibid.* 14 (Vol. 10), p. 142-143.
26. *Ibid.*, p. 123.
27. Hahnemann S. *Materia Medica Pura.* New Delhi, India: B. Jain Publishers;2002: 616-617.
28. *Ibid.*, p. 624.
29. Kent J. *Lectures on Materia Medica*. New Delhi, India: B. Jain Publishers;1993: 954.
30. *Ibid.*, p. 973.
31. *Ibid.* 14 (Vol. 3), p. 162.
32. *Ibid.,* p. 221.
33. *Ibid. 29*, p. 315-316.
34. *Ibid.*, p. 323.

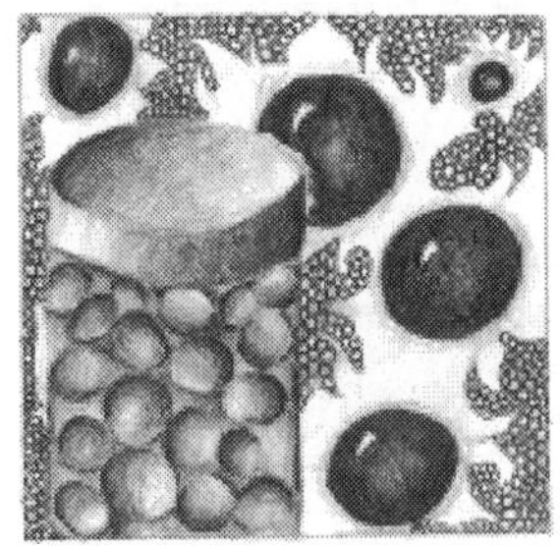

6 - Repertorization

Repertories are indexes of proving symptoms, organized by body part.

By the time your veterinarian is ready to begin searching for the curative remedy, she has spent considerable time and energy understanding your animal's case. She has elicited all of the patient's symptoms from you and your animal's health records, discovered which symptoms are complete and which are concomitants, carefully teased out all the possible modalities for each symptom, highlighted general, mental, and peculiar symptoms, and placed all of them on the patient's timeline. To your homeopath (as to you), your companion is unique, even in a practice with hundreds of patients.

I do not recommend treating your own animals, but I have included this chapter to familiarize you with the process of selecting the curative remedy. You may find it useful to know exactly how remedies are selected. Read this chapter as if you are working the cases yourself.

Repertorization is the process of selecting the remedy that covers the most rubrics, or symptoms, of the patient. The word "repertory" means repository, or storehouse. In this case, the storehouse is for symptoms and their associated remedies. Repertories are the index for all the symptoms of each remedy, ordered by the part of the body in which the symptom is expressed. These symptoms are derived from provings, and recorded in materia medicas. (For more on provings, refer back to the chapter What Does Homeopathy Heal?)

Another source of remedy information is poisoning reports. For example, arsenic (undiluted) has been used as a poison, and the study of death reports and records from attendant physicians provide data as to the effects of this particular chemical on the human body. One famous poisoning was that of Socrates, who was put to death using hemlock, or conium, which is a homeopathic remedy (after being highly diluted). Before dying, Socrates suffered from an ascending paralysis (starting in the feet and moving upwards), which means that this remedy could potentially be helpful in similar conditions, such as in canine degenerative myelopathy (progressive paralysis beginning in the tail and hind legs and working up the spinal cord).

The materia medica of conium, derived from reports such as this, states, "Sensation of weakness even to trembling, in right thigh while walking. Staggering gait. Painless loss of power in lower limbs; faltering, vacillating gait; staggers as if drunk, dragging his legs after him."[1] Notice how the observable symptom is listed, not the diagnosis. This makes the rubrics more specific as to how disease is expressed in the individual patient, rather than describing the symptoms common to a certain diagnosis. From these symptoms, rubrics were derived and put into the repertory. Conium is found in rubrics such as stumbling when walking, incoordination, and numbness of the legs, for example. This remedy is also found in rubrics describing ataxia, which is a lack of awareness of where the limbs are in space. Ataxic animals walk as if they are drunk. The flow of information looks like this:

• • •

provings or poisonings >> materia medicas >> repertories

• • •

In the repertory, the rubrics, or symptoms, are listed in alphabetical order within their respective body parts. This makes them easy to find while working up a case. Once the key symptoms of the patient have been selected (as discussed in the Case Analysis chapter) they are matched with the most descriptive rubric. After this methodical process is complete, the purely mechanical work of discovering which remedies show up in the most rubrics can begin. It's a Venn diagram, on a very large scale.

The main repertory used for the cases in this book is the *New World Veterinary Repertory* (*NWVR*), developed by myself and my co-author Dr. Richard Pitcairn, specifically for use by veterinary homeopaths. (For an excellent description of the historical development of the repertory, read Dr. Pitcairn's preface in the *NWVR*.) There are computer programs that make repertorization much easier. (See the references at the back of this book.) Once the desired rubrics are selected, the software program does the legwork and quickly provides a chart showing which remedies are in which rubrics. However, if you are going to study homeopathy, don't start at the computer. Spend your first years reading through the repertory chapters and finalizing your selections in the textbook. Use the computer only to create your final repertorization chart, as a time-saver. Work by hand until the rubrics in the repertory become as familiar as old friends. This has many advantages to any homeopath's skill development, and the results will be carried with you. As a new homeopath, you will find yourself learning the layout of the repertory better if you've been holding the hard copy, and your accuracy in rubric selection will develop more quickly this way.

After carefully selecting the best rubrics for the case, the final step is to list each remedy for each patient rubric and find out which remedies are common to the greatest number of rubrics. Usually, the curative remedy will be found near the top of this list, since these remedies are the ones found in most of the rubrics. Even if you work from a textbook to enhance your knowledge of the repertory, this last mechanical step is easily performed on the computer program. For those who prefer completing their analysis by hand, a partial example of a hand repertorization chart is found in the References at the end of the book, as well as a link to a complete pdf chart online.

Why a Book is Better

There are many advantages to beginning the repertorization of the patient with a book rather than a computer program. You get to know your tool, the repertory, much quicker. The mind learns faster when the sections of study are related spatially. For example, you begin to hold in your mind the layout of the chapter on coughing, and where the section describing inciting factors sits on the page. You note from the printed word that the inciting section is quite long and intricate, and thus with your next coughing patient, you spend more time discovering exactly what aggravates this particular patient's cough. For the next patient, while you are paging through the respiratory section, studying the aggravations, you happily discover another section called "impeded by." The topography of the book naturally lends itself to study, and during the process, the book becomes more familiar and you become a better homeopath.

By contrast, in a computer listing, each section looks exactly like any other section. Your mind's eye view of the repertory changes according to how you have arranged the page on your computer screen, with the chapter title on the top and the sub-sections either open or closed. A great tool, but not for developing familiarity with its contents.

Memory is a visual process.

A book enriches your memory as your eyes scan the pages, examining which sections are longer, which rubrics have less remedies (and thus are more specific), and sub-sections which have more intricate descriptions that may prove useful in that next patient. You can page through and compare one chapter to another, discovering what is unique about the Expectoration chapter and what makes up the Chill, Cold chapter. You might find the perfect rubric in one section, but discover quickly that it has too few remedies, and thus would be very limiting in some cases. Other rubrics may stand out immediately in the book as being way too inclusive, presenting hundreds of remedies instead of a select few dozen. The mind remembers the look of the section better than it might remember the number listed in the computer.

Many times I have discovered the rubric most exactly describing my patient's symptom just by perusing the pertinent chapter and bumping into it on my way to the page I at first had in mind. The visual image of each page stays longer in my mind than the printed words themselves, thus giving me a leg-up when I pass through that chapter the next time. Interestingly, the work to match the patient with the remedy may also have a visual component, as you "see" the patient and you "see" the remedy in the same part of the brain that is seeing the repertory's pages. This visually-oriented sensory memory works best with the static layout of a book.

That said, there is absolutely no match to the computer once you have finished your rubric selection. Often I begin with the book, finalize my rubric selection, and only then turn to the computer to produce my final repertorization chart. For example, I selected the following rubrics from the book (the number following each rubric reflects the number of remedies in that rubric):

Sleep; during; snoring (34)
Generalities; agg.; touch; slight (13)
Face; proper; twitching (68)

Then, rather than listing all the remedies by hand and laboriously counting out which ones are common to more than one rubric, I turn to the computer repertory and print up a nice chart like this:

	bell.	nux-v.	ign.	chin.	op.	acon.
Analysis	100	96	76	59	50	49
Sleep; During; snoring	3	3	1	3	4	
Generalities; Agg.; Touch; slight	4	4	2	4		4
Face; Proper; Twitching	4	3	2		4	1

The rubrics are in the left column, under "Analysis." The remedies are abbreviated across the top row. In the computer, this chart would proceed to the right until all the remedies are listed. You can quickly and easily see which remedies occur in all three rubrics (bell., nux-v., and ign.), and three which have two of the rubrics (chin., op., and acon.). (The numbers under the remedies are discussed next.) This is a quick way to select remedies that might fit your particular patient. Truly a joy to use in these final stages of your study. With a computer, you can also navigate quickly to cross-references (related rubrics), rather than having to page through to another chapter. You can also customize the page, leaving out remedies entirely as you study the rubrics, or leaving out sub-sections if you prefer reading only major headings. Of course, changing the color and font is another personal touch not offered by the printed page.

Remedy Grading

In the chart above, the numbers inside the boxes refer to the remedy grade. This is the frequency with which that symptom has been reported by the respective provers. For example, many provers who took belladonna (bell.) reported facial twitching, represented by the number 4, but this symptom was only rarely reported by provers taking aconite (acon.), thus earning the number 1. In the printed repertory, the remedy grade is indicated by different typefaces. Grade 1 is plain type (calc), grade 2 italicized (*calc*), grade 3 bolded (**calc**), and in some repertories grade four is all capitals (CALC). Remedies with a higher grade are more important in the rubric, because they have been seen more frequently by provers taking the medicine. If that particular symptom is strong in the patient, the curative remedy is likely to have a similar strength in the same symptom.

The row labeled "Analysis" weights the remedies according to their grade and presence in each rubric. In this chart, belladonna was present in all the rubrics, and had the highest sum total of the grades. So belladonna, with one 3 grading and two 4 gradings, is assigned the highest analysis number, 100. Next comes nux vomica, with 96% of the total as compared to belladonna, since nux, though present in all the rubrics as well, had two 3 gradings but only one 4 grading. The analysis number quickly shows which remedy is most strongly represented among the selected rubrics, and how the following remedies compare. When completing the repertorization chart by hand, simply add the grades within each column to get the relative strength for each remedy.

Organization of the Repertory

The repertory is divided into chapters according to the part of the body, beginning with the mind and head and moving down through the chest and abdomen, all the way to the feet. These are the chapters in the *NWVR:*

Mind
Vertigo
Head, Internal
Head, External
Eyes
Vision
Ears
Hearing
Nose
Face
Mouth
Teeth
External Throat
Stomach
Abdomen
Rectum
Stool
Urinary
Urine
Prostate
Genitalia
Male
Female
Larynx
Respiration
Cough
Expectoration
Chest
Back
Extremities, Anterior (front limbs)
Extremities, Posterior (rear limbs)

Sleep
Cold
Fever
Perspiration
Skin
Circulation
Generalities

There are myriad ways for the body to express illness. The chapters mirror this complexity. For example, the headings within the Cough chapter begin like this:

COUGH
GENERAL (119)
TIME
AGGRAVATION
AMELIORATION
CONCOMITANTS (106)
Anxious (4)
Asthmatic, wheezy (17)
Barking (40)
Cachectic (with progressive weight loss) (4)
Catarrhal (inflammation of mucous membranes) (32)
Choking (27)
Chronic (14)
Clear, ringing (5)
Clock, like tick of, in its regularity (1)
Concussive, shaking, shattering (37)
Consciousness, loss of, with (3)
.......(the chapter continues)

The chapter begins with time, aggravation, and amelioration, thus making it easy to find the modalities for the case under study. Modalities, as studied in the chapter Case Analysis, are vital to characterizing the uniqueness of the symptom for each particular patient. The numbers in parentheses refer to the number of remedies in each rubric. (Headings without numbers, such as Aggravation or Amelioration, only have remedies within their sub-sections, which are not listed here.) This is what you would see on the computer screen with only the first level of rubrics selected, which is the easier way to navigate without being overwhelmed by the pure number of lines. However, as a new homeopath using a computer, with this view, you would miss the incredible complexity of the Concomitant rubric. Written below are the first few sub-rubrics under Concomitants, listing all the symptoms which can occur at the same time as the cough, or the locations which suffer from symptoms at the same time as the cough:

COUGH; CONCOMITANTS
Abdomen (1)
Abdominal pain (bellyache) (25)
Air hunger (trying to get air) (1)
Anxiety, fear (8)
Cheeks, drawing in (1)
Constipation (1)
Convulsions, spasms, with (17)
Coryza (2)
Crying out (8)
Dizziness (vertigo) (6)
Doubling up (1)
Emaciation (4)
Erections (1)
Eructations (7)
Exhaustion after coughing (4)
Extremities, anterior, pain in (2)
Falling to the ground (1)
Fever, during (79)
Flatus, discharged up and down (1)
Frightened (2)
Front limbs, pain in (2)
.......(the chapter continues)

....and it goes on and on! This wonderful section might be missed entirely when clicking through the computer, whereas in the book, it would be right there in front of you. Make your books old friends before you reach for those computer repertories. The extra effort will reward you with greater accuracy in your prescriptions.

• • •

Now let's look at another case from my practice:

Joy, the Lame Airedale Dog

Joy is a four year-old spayed female terrier, who had been lame for two years. Her favorite sport of ball chasing was becoming increasingly difficult. Here is her timeline, so that you have a better sense of her case before studying her symptoms:

Joy's timeline:

5/05	birth
9/05	smelly ears; later fell off a rock wall, then off the deck
12/05	spayed
3/06	mucus strings when urinating, licking the area
11/06	discharge from left eye, red sclera and conjunctiva, rubbing eye
1/07	refusing to go upstairs; then lameness began
1/08	lameness continued; bloody diarrhea after a non-steroidal anti-inflammatory drug
7/08	inflammation in right ear
10/08	tender to palpation of neck, back muscles, and left front biceps tendon; laser treatment
11/08	conjunctivitis in right eye; easy startling in sleep began, maybe dreams began?
10/09	began treatment with homeopathy

• • •

See how her lameness problem begins subtly, with Joy refusing to go upstairs? The timeline also depicts other symptoms she experienced as a younger dog. All of these, her eye and ear symptoms, and trouble in the urinary tract, all resolved as she got older. These symptoms have not been cured, only receding into the background as her lameness worsened. We would expect these symptoms to return as she responded to the correct remedy. Here is her complete symptom list:

Joy's symptom list:

startles easily, especially to light touch, more prominent recently
    if touched in sound sleep leaps up "as if to run away"
sleeps late
dreams a lot: runs in sleep, vocalizes, rolls eyes
left front leg lameness worse after exercise; stiff
mucousy grey eye discharge
    history of red swollen conjunctiva in right eye
brown odorous wax in both ears, but worse on the left
history of mucus strings from vulva when urinating
    mucosa very red
as pup bowel movements "hard to pick up"
    mucus coating (clear white and slimy)
    second bowel movement looser
    straining after finished "as if more was in there"
    increased urgency
vaccinated regularly

• • •

Match the rubrics to the patient, not the patient to the rubrics.

It is critical to develop your complete symptom list before cracking open the repertory. The picture of the patient must be firm in your mind (and in your homeopath's mind) before you begin reading rubrics. If you page through rubrics looking to find your patient, then you will be matching your case to the index of rubrics rather than matching rubrics to the patient's symptoms. This is a subtle yet powerful distinction. For example, if I just know my patient coughs a lot in the morning, I might select Cough; morning (80). But after careful study, I develop a strong clear picture of the patient that is based on what I see, not on what is listed in the book. So I know that my patient is most troubled and anxious by coughing that occurs just when he begins to move in the morning. These rubrics are very suitable, and most exactly describe my patient: Cough; concomitant; anxiety, fear (8); and Cough; agg.; waking, on (64). See the difference? Know your patient, *then* find her rubrics.

"It is a capital mistake to theorize before one has data. Insensibly one begins to twist facts to suit theories, instead of theories to suit facts."—Sherlock Holmes [2]

Now let's repertorize Joy. At the beginning of her case, I used the remedy sulfur, repeated every few weeks, with slow improvement. Finally, this remedy no longer helped. She kept slipping back. I was palliating. At this point in the case young Joy is described by the client as, "A stiff old dog who is crippled with arthritis, stiff and gimpy as if wearing hobbles." So even though the remedy did act, and she was clearly better after each dose, she was not well. This is the time to re-evaluate her entire case and search for a more fitting remedy.

The first step during a re-evaluation is to be sure you have not missed any information about the patient. Then re-match the symptoms with the most apt rubrics. So for "startles easily, especially to light touch...if touched in sound sleep leaps up 'as if to run away,'" I found Mind; startled easily (98). A very close match for part of the symptom. Then I searched in the Sleep chapter to find a description of her startling during sleep. I found Sleep;

during; starting up (as in a fright) (81). Perfect. So next I have "sleeps late," but this symptom is not particularly descriptive of Joy and her lameness. "Dreams a lot, runs in sleep, vocalizes, eyes roll," is more interesting. Barking and moving her eyes very likely indicates dreaming. So the rubric Sleep; restless; from many dreams (63) seems just right. (This is from the Boenninghausen repertory listed at the end of the book.) Regarding her lameness, the word "stiff" is not very descriptive—are they just stiff, or also sore? Difficult to be sure. So I'll leave that symptom out of the repertorization and just check for lameness symptoms in the materia medica for confirmation once I select the remedy. The closest description to cover her mucousy grey eye discharge and red swollen conjunctiva was Eyes; proper; inflammation (74).

Moving down the list, Joy often had a mucoid discharge, whether from her eyes, her urinary tract, or her stools. Remember that symptoms referring to the whole body (generalities) are more useful for finding the proper remedy, and that particular symptoms occurring in many locations can be generalized? So this rubric fit: Generalities; discharge; increased, slimy (102). For her ears, I liked Ears; earwax; secretion, increased (34) as the most specific rubric. As a veterinarian, it helps to have seen many many cases of ear conditions. From experience, I know that the material described in her ears was excess wax, and not an infection. Then finally comes "bowel movements 'hard to pick up,' mucus coating (clear white and slimy), second bowel movement looser, straining after finished 'as if more was in there,' increased urgency." The most peculiar aspect of this symptom complex is the coating, which is described in rubric language as Stool; mucus, of; covered with (39).

This discussion is meant to give you an idea of what your homeopath will be doing with the information you have provided. There are many possible rubrics, and careful thinking goes into each selection. Study the recommended books in the References at the end of this book if you would like to familiarize yourself more fully with the intricate world of rubric selection.

• • •

Here is the chart of our selected rubrics:

	phos.	sulf.	sep.	nit-ac.	puls.	petr.	bell.	kali-c.
Analysis	100	100	97	91	87	87	77	75
Mind; Startled easily	4	3	3	2		3	4	4
Sleep; During; starting up	3	4	4	3	4	3	4	2
Sleep; Restless; from many dreams	1	2	1	1	3	2		3
Eyes; Proper; Inflammation	4	4	4	2	4	2	4	
Generalities; Discharge; increased, slimy	4	4	3	2	4	1	3	2
Ears; Earwax; secretion, increased	2	1	1	3	4	1	1	4
Stool; Mucus, of; covered with	1	1	2	2	3	1	1	1

As you can see, there are four remedies which are found in all of the rubrics: phos., sulf., sep., and nit-ac. The next step is to go to the source (materia medica) and read about those particular remedies. Sulfur was used before in her case, without curative action, so we can rule it out. I will not go into the materia medica of phosph. and nit-ac., as they are not what helped Joy, and the discussion is beyond the scope of this book, but I will describe sepia so that you can see how close it is to her symptoms. In my study I examined each top remedy, and some not so near the top, in order to be certain of my choice. If you study the top remedies and they do not match the patient, go back and examine your rubrics to find closer matches.

• • •

Joy's materia medica:

I left out materia medica referring to specific dreams, because we don't know what Joy is chasing when she sleeps. But it's a sure bet that she is dreaming, since she is moving and vocalizing during sleep. Most importantly, the client mentioned this on her own without prompting, so this symptom becomes more important to the case. Voluntarily submitted information often proves more accurate and important than data gained only after much detailed questioning.

sepia:
Mind: Nerves very sensitive to the least noise.[3]
Sleep: Twitching of limbs.[4]
Upper Limbs: Pain as from dislocation in shoulder joint after exertion. Paralytic drawing and tearing in arm and armpit to fingers. Lameness and falling asleep of arms and fingers....Stiffness of elbow and wrist joints.[5]
Stool: ...stools difficult, covered with mucus....terrible straining to pass stool, which is covered with mucus....[6]
Nerves: Twitching of limbs during sleep.[7]
Sleep: Twitching of limbs.[8]
Eyes: ...eyes agglutinated in morning....redness of conjunctiva....[9]
Urinary Organs: ...urine...cloudy and dark, as if mixed with mucus....[10]
Kent: ...stool covered with a great quantity of jelly-like mucus....[11]

• • •

Sepia looks very like Joy. There is the peculiar covering of mucus over the stools, the movement during sleep, and symptoms in the upper limbs which match Joy's lameness. Also read about redness in the eyes, and suspected mucus in the urine. All Joy's symptoms.

• • •

After receiving a single dose of sepia 200C, Joy's lameness came and went for a period of time. But by two weeks after the dose, she had "only a very slight hitch." The client, for the first time, noted that exercise would actually improve her lameness. This is a hallmark of sepia, which was not clear at the intake consultation. Three months later, her eyes were wet, and the right side was worse, just like when she had had these symptoms three years before. This return of old symptoms was a very happy sign of a good remedy match. Her eyes cleared up on their own without treatment.

Joy's ear and urinary troubles did not return over the course of her treatment. Is this cause for worry? Not necessarily. Often once the patient is feeling better, old symptom recurrences can be so brief and innocuous that client and patient hardly notice them before they disappear again.

Joy needed two more doses of remedy over the following eight months. As of this publication, well over three years after her last dose, she remains a "healthy, happy dog." She gets up "with delight" even as early as 5:30 am, no longer sleeping in. She occasionally has clear gel in her eyes, no problems with urination or defecation, she still twitches and vocalizes in her sleep but not every day, her weight is perfect, her startling is not too bad, and her ears are only slightly waxy. May she live on to a ripe old age chasing that beloved ball!

• • •

Now you have experienced a taste of the work involved after the intake consult is complete. This chapter highlights the importance of careful objective complete symptom descriptions. With an excellent base of accurate symptoms, the case will be easier to study and the patient will experience the best outcome possible.

• • •

Chapter 6 References

1. Hering C. *The Guiding Symptoms of Our Materia Medica*. Vol. 4. Paharganj, New Delhi, India: B. Jain Publishers;1995: 430 - 431.
2. Doyle, Arthur Conan. "A Scandal in Bohemia." N.p.: n.p., n.d. N. pag. *East of the Web Short Stories*. Web. 11 Sept. 2015. <http://www.eastoftheweb.com/short-stories/UBooks/ScanBohe.shtml>.
3. *Ibid.* 1 (Vol. 9), p. 298.
4. *Ibid.*, p. 342.
5. *Ibid.*, p. 335 – 336.
6. *Ibid.*, p. 318 – 319.
7. *Ibid.*, p. 340.
8. *Ibid.*, p. 342.
9. *Ibid.*, p. 306.
10. *Ibid.*, p. 320.
11. Kent J. *Lectures on Materia Medica*. New Delhi, India: B. Jain Publishers;1993: 922.

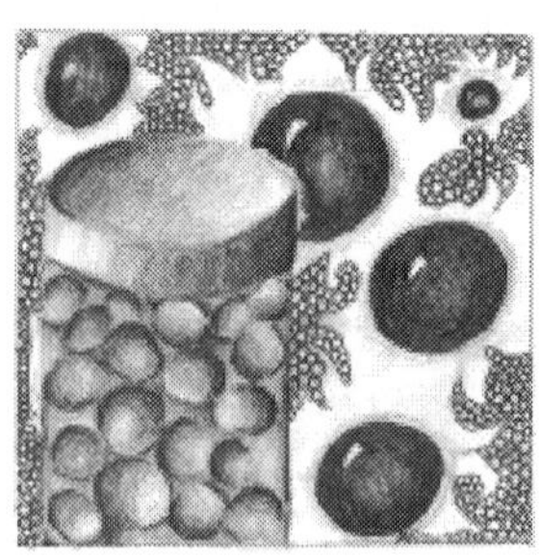

7 - Posology

Potency Selection—The Final Step

Having decided on the remedy, the next and final step facing your veterinarian is potency selection. While you will not have to make this decision, nor help your homeopath, this chapter has been included for the sake of completeness, and to answer questions for the curious. Often the loudest detractors against homeopathy focus on the dilute nature of its medicines, so having an understanding of this aspect is important.

What is potency? It refers to the strength of the remedy, or how much power has been developed through the processes of dilution and succussion, as discussed in the chapter The Basics. Just as the selection of remedy must match the symptoms of the patient, likewise the potency must match the strength of the vital force. In other words, the power needed to bend a blade of grass is different than the power needed to shake an ancient pine. Many homeopaths consider the selection of potency more difficult than that of the remedy itself!

What does the *Organon* have to say about the matter? A. 278: "Now the question arises what this ideal degree of smallness is, the degree that is certain and gentle in its remedial effect: how small should the dose of a given correctly chosen homoeopathic medicine be to cure a case of disease in the best way?"[1]

This surely gets your attention, doesn't it? Asking how *small* the dose should be instead of how *large* it needs to be to overcome a symptom nicely encapsulates the difference between allopathic and homeopathic medicine.

As you recall in the chapter The Basics, homeopathic medicines are prepared through dilution and succussion, thus freeing up the healing energy of the substances so that it is available to the patient. The patient, you might also remember, is sick on the energetic plane, so this is where the medicine must be directed. As the medicines are diluted more and more, they become stronger and stronger; their medicinal power, or potency, developed to a higher and higher degree.

The more the remedy is diluted and succussed, the stronger it becomes.

A. 278 continued: "To solve this problem, to determine for a given medicine used in homoeopathic practice what dose would be sufficient and at the same time small enough to effect the gentlest, quickest cure, is not a matter of theoretical conjecture, as one can easily understand. Theorizing and specious sophistry cannot enlighten us on this subject, nor can every possible eventuality be tabulated in advance. Only pure experiment, the meticulous observation of the sensitivity of each patient, and sound experience can determine this in each individual case."[2]

What is Hahnemann saying here? What is 'specious sophistry'? According to Webster, sophistry is "subtly deceptive reasoning or argumentation."[3] Hahnemann is reminding us that we can't just decide that a certain dose is correct for all cases of disease before us. We can't make a table with all the contingencies on one side and the correct potency on the other side, for convenient and sure-fire reference. No, the correct dose must be decided individually for each separate patient—for each unique presentation of disease. It's not a simple matter of how many grams of drug per pound of patient. The correct dose is determined by the strength of the vital force and the development of the disease which is unbalancing that particular vital force. Selecting the proper potency of the remedy is just as important as selecting the right remedy.

A. 278 continued: "It would be foolish to disregard what pure experience teaches us about the smallness of the dose necessary for homoeopathic cure and to favor the large doses of the inappropriate (allopathic) medicines of the old school, which do not homoeopathically affect the sick part of the organism, but only attack the part that the disease has not taken hold of."[4]

This describes what happens when medicines are given that do not match the disease picture of the patient. By definition, a medicine which does not match the disease state must overlap onto the non-diseased part of the organism (the parts not yet expressing symptoms). The body reacts to these in a non-curative fashion, and modern medicine calls these reactions "side effects." But when a homeopathic remedy is given, and when its strength matches the strength of the illness, a deep healing response results.

A. 279: "Pure experience *absolutely* proves that even in a chronic or complicated disease, when there is no extensive damage to some vital organ, and though all other foreign medicinal influence has been withheld from the patient, *the dose of the highly potentized homoeopathic remedy beginning the treatment of a significant (chronic) disease can, as a rule, not be made so small*

that it is not stronger than the natural disease,

that it cannot at least partially overcome it,

that it cannot at least partially extinguish it in the feelings of the vital principle,

that it cannot start the process of cure."[5]

So no matter how dilute the dose is, it always has an effect on the vital force. So what are the considerations your veterinarian makes in order to select the proper potency? There are many factors, but they all center upon matching the potency to the degree to which the disease has impinged upon the patient's vital force. Like a fist into a rubber ball, this impingement depends both upon the strength of the fist (disease) and the firmness of the rubber (vital force). It's not a linear relationship, but more a web of influences, interacting over time. Consider how firmly the fist was clenched, how fast the fist was traveling before hitting the ball, how much power the arm behind the fist contained, whether the ball was moving before it was struck, the pliability of the ball's material, whether the strike was dead on or a glancing blow....all these factors determine the effect of this impact. Your veterinarian must consider a complicated set of variables before deciding on the proper potency.

Here's another analogy to describe potency. Picture trying to push a stranded truck on a flat surface. No matter how hard you shove on the side door, that truck is not going to move. You have to line up your power with the orientation of the wheels. You first get in the cab and turn the steering wheel to align the front tires with the rear ones. Then you check to be sure the brakes are off, and the truck is in neutral. You might gather some friends to help. Finally, you all apply your most powerful shoves together, at the same time, directly behind the truck. It's moving! You successfully followed the principles of potency selection. You set up the proper conditions, then applied the power, right where it would have the most effect. Selecting potencies is a lot like this. By studying the patient, your veterinarian will be able to select just the right power to get that truck rolling. Once it starts to slow down, then another push is needed, and the patient is ready for the next dose. "Force, to be effective, must be supplied not only in the proper amount, but in the proper direction and at the proper time."[6]

. . .

Dr. Close gives us five considerations important to the selection of potency [7]:

susceptibility of the patient
seat of the disease
nature and intensity of the disease
stage and duration of the disease
previous treatment of the disease

. . .

Susceptibility

What is susceptibility? Let's start with Webster: "Lack of ability to resist some extraneous agent; sensitivity."[8] How susceptible is the truck to your push? How hard do you have to exert yourself to get it moving? Maybe the truck has rusted wheels, or is sitting in mud, or perhaps pointing slightly up a hill. You would need to push harder. But what if it's already pointing down a slope? If the potency is too large and the patient very susceptible, then the case may spin out of control, aggravating excessively. You might run the truck into a river. If the potency is too small, the effect might be negligible, leading you and your veterinarian into the search for a new remedy, when actually all that is needed is a higher potency of the same remedy. In a nutshell, susceptibility refers to how much the correct remedy will affect the patient. Keep in mind, however, that this is not a static quality in the patient. Susceptibility can vary over time.

• • •

Susceptibility is highest in the following patients:

young vigorous animals
animals with greater vitality
sensitive nervous patients
animals without pathology
patients who have NOT received a lot of (non-curative) medicines in the past (exception in the next paragraph)
patients in healthy environments
  good food, limited vaccinations—or none
  appropriate and regular exercise
  a stable loving predictable home
patients with certain diseases
  higher susceptibility in patients with seizures
  lower susceptibility in heart valve disease
  (this also relates to the seat of the disease, described below)

• • •

In general, the patients described above will do very well with higher potencies. Where there is a rule, however, there are always exceptions. For example, a patient who has received a lot of drugs, who might require low potencies as their susceptibility has been exhausted, may only respond to the higher potencies as a sort of a "wake-up" to their beleaguered vital force. This may depend on the strength of their vital force (which is different than their susceptibility). This overdosed patient would do well with a higher potency, such as 30C or higher. "Allowance should be made, however, for the varying ability of examiners. One man, keen of perception, will see many things in a case which another not so endowed will fail to see."[9] Selection of the potency is an art, not a science.

• • •

Here's a chart to illustrate the relationship between susceptibility, strength of vital force, and suitable potency of the medicine:

Strength of Vital Force
High

High Potency or Low Potency with frequent repetitions Susceptibility	High Potency Susceptibility
Low Low Potency	High Low Potency with infrequent repetitions

Low
Strength of Vital Force

Susceptibility is a difficult concept to master. It measures both how reactive the patient might be to the curative remedy, but also how much of a strong push the patient can take. So a highly susceptible patient with a strong vital force would be able to progress more quickly towards cure with a higher potency, or a single strong push, whereas a highly susceptible patient with a weak vital force would benefit more from the gentle push of a lower potency, given infrequently.

Seat of the Disease

This refers to the location of the symptoms in the body. As mentioned in the discussion of susceptibility, a patient with serious disease manifesting in the heart would probably do better with lower potencies, whereas one with neurological symptoms may need higher potencies. Neurological symptoms such as tremors and memory loss don't have the same potential for disaster with aggravations, whereas an aggravation in a patient with a heart condition could very well be fatal. If the skin is the most diseased area, then the practitioner may well look to other factors when choosing potency, as both high and low potencies could potentially be helpful.

Nature and Intensity of the Disease

This is Dr. Close's third consideration for potency selection. How bad is the patient's disease? With itching but no skin eruptions, a higher potency might be recommended, whereas a patient with skin ulcers might do better with a lower potency. The vital force which has allowed ulcers on the skin is weaker and has a stronger disease than the vital force that simply itches. In another situation, a dog with debilitating diarrhea may need a lower potency than one with occasional loose stools.

Stage and Duration of the Disease

How long has your animal been sick? Older animals who have spent years suffering from their complaints might respond better to lower potencies, like gentle nudges, until they begin reacting and feeling better.

Younger animals with relatively recent symptoms will do better with higher potencies.

Previous Treatment of the Disease

Finally, as alluded to before, patients with extensive non-curative treatment (of any type) may be weak and confused. The vital force reacts to any medicine given, whether it is curative or not, and this reaction takes energy and focus. When the medicine matches some symptoms but is contrary to others, the vital force cannot work in a clear, focused manner. An organized, coherent reaction, as required in the curative process, is impossible. Patients who have taken medications frequently or for prolonged periods respond better to lower potencies. Giving a high potency in these situations would be similar to shoving really hard on a truck stuck in the mud. You will just crumple the bumper! The over-medicated patient's vital force is jaded and sluggish, unable to react curatively to a sudden single push. On the other hand, always keep in mind that the vital force and its interaction with the curative remedy is not a single-line continuum. As discussed above, many suppressed patients actually need a high potency to get them reacting again, like using a tractor to get the stuck truck out of the mud. There are multiple interacting factors which determine the path of healing after a remedy dose. Your veterinarian wrestles with all of these questions when determining the proper potency.

This quote is attributed to Dr. Guernsey, a homeopathic physician of obstetrics who practiced in Philadelphia in the mid-to-late 1800's [10]: "A skillful artist may indeed construct a harmony with the various vibrations of the same chord; but what a more beautiful and perfect harmony might be construct[ed] by a proper combination of all the sounds that can be elicited from his instrument."[11] Veterinarians comfortable with all potencies will be more successful than those who limit their dispensing to only a few.

• • •

Now let's look at the cases we have been following, to watch potencies in action. Wilkins the dove, described in the chapter What Does Homeopathy Heal? started off with an X potency. I prescribed this potency twice daily, for three reasons. One was that I had it in my house call bag. Two was that he was an elderly patient with a very active uncomfortable condition (straining to produce droppings). If this condition didn't resolve, he could die, so I needed both a gentle nudge, but a persistent one. Repeating a low potency seemed to ease him and get him moving into a stronger state, at which time he was ready for the 200C dose. Over his lifetime, he received a few more doses of the same remedy at increasing potencies, widely spaced.

Ronnie the squirrel was in a similar situation, elderly, and also in a serious acute situation that had come on quickly. I began with a single dose of a 30X potency, not wanting to repeat as I could not see her remedy state clearly. After her subsequent continued decline, an additional symptom led me to another remedy. After three doses of the 30X potency, she not only recovered her former vitality, but returned to a level of health she had not seen for the past full year. She responded so well that it was clear she did not need a higher potency to follow.

Unfortunately, I have no record of Thomas' potency, but Ida, the cat who had been sneezing bloody pus for the previous year, had a single 30C dose. Even though he was an older cat at twelve years, his vital force was strong enough to limit his disease to this symptom, despite repeated bouts of antibiotics. I might have gone higher than 30C if he was younger or if his symptoms were more violently expressed. 30C fit him perfectly, however, as evidenced by his aggravation after the dose (he began rubbing his nose and sneezing feverishly, and this lasted a few days), followed by a complete resolution of his symptoms. He did not need another dose for the entire next year.

Solly, the cat with a urinary blockage, was introduced in the chapter The Basics. I began with 30X because he also needed something on an emergency basis and that remedy was on hand. Meanwhile, his positive reaction gave the guardian time to pick up 30C, a good potency for a patient in a critical condition who had responded well to 30X. Jumping to

30C was easier than trying to find a 100X or 200X (not so readily available), and this jump served Solly well. Months later, a 200C resolved a minor recurrence of his disease. As demonstrated by this case, sometimes the potency is predicated upon what is on hand, and the vital force rises to the occasion. An LM potency would also have been helpful in Solly's case, especially since he was on allopathic medications. LM potencies are very helpful to use when slowly weaning off palliative medicines.

Ruthie, the young dog with post-surgical illness and severe constipation, needed only one dose of 30C. Acute conditions respond more rapidly to homeopathy than to allopathic medications, so they are a great way to showcase the power of this medicine. Ruthie had no aggravation, indicating that the potency of the remedy exactly matched the strength of her disease. In any case, in acute diseases the remedy aggravation may be very small. Read A. 157: "But however certain it is that a homoeopathically chosen remedy, because of its appropriateness and the minuteness of the dose, gently removes and destroys its analogous *acute* disease without manifesting its remaining unhomoeopathic symptoms, i.e., without arousing any new significant complaints, it is nevertheless usual (but only when the dose is not appropriately attenuated) for it to effect some *small* aggravation in the first hour or first few hours after it is taken and for several hours if the dose is rather too large."[12] So with the small ("attenuated") doses given in homeopathic treatment, a patient may be cured of his acute illness with only a very small aggravation. That's called hitting the bull's eye! Small aggravations may be easy to miss. In Ruthie's case, she might have had briefly increased abdominal pain, mild and undetectable to anyone but Ruthie. We may also miss aggravations if they occur in the mental or emotional sphere, or if they happen while we are away at work.

Next there is Hogarth, the Labrador with a persistent bloody nasal discharge from The Intake Consultation chapter. Hogarth is a middle-aged patient with a severe problem. As evidenced by his history of "arthritis" bad enough that he had trouble navigating stairs, Hogarth's disease had not limited itself to one body system. This patient would not do well with a very high potency, because his vital force is simply not strong enough to rise to the challenge and match that level of power. And yet the slow steady deterioration he had experienced over the past months called for a slow steady yet powerful remedy. In Hogarth's case, the LM potencies came highly recommended, with their ability to be flexible according to the needs of the case (remedies given in water have this advantage), yet the power to arrest a long steady decline in an aging vital force. LM's are unique among potencies in that though highly diluted, they can be extremely gentle, due to their method of preparation. Hogarth might also have done well with a 30C. In every case, the practitioner must always be in the habit of paying close attention to the state of the patient before repeating a remedy, even with the LM potencies. Hogarth responded well to widely-spaced doses.

Also in The Intake Consultation chapter is Charlie the Bernese Mountain Dog with itching and gulping. Here we have a young dog, barely two years old, and a recent problem. However, take note that the recent problem comes on top of lifelong emotional concerns having to do with fear and anxiety over being touched, riding in the car, and sounds, as well as an excessive reaction to pain. So even though he's a young dog, his disease has become firmly entrenched in both the physical, mental, and emotional planes. If an excessively high potency had been used, Charlie would have had the potential to aggravate quite severely. So what would be the proper potency for a young strong animal with moderate disease in multiple planes? I began with 30C, and nearly two months later he required a 200C dose when his symptoms began creeping back. In Charlie's case, I could probably have started with a higher potency, since his only detectable aggravation was some very "stinky" poops a few days after the 30C dose. But with his explosive potential (emotionally), I did not want to risk beginning too high. Two days after the 200C potency, he had a day of increased whining and restlessness, "humping" everything, and general malaise. This resolved quickly, and he steadily improved on all levels until he was described as doing "awesomely." Often the first remedy in a new patient "lines up" the symptoms so that they respond more quickly and smoothly to subsequent doses, given when indicated. Avoiding large jumps in potencies has served me well in my practice.

Moving on to the chapter Repertorization, we find Joy, the chronically lame four year-old Airedale Terrier. The client told me, "When she's running she's beautiful," and that she was "a happy dog, full of joy." But all this had changed with her lameness. In spite of multiple different types of treatments over the past two years, her lameness had persisted. Joy could no longer keep up on a run with her caretaker. Her favorite sport of ball chasing was a thing of the past. My client was seriously considering euthanasia. Joy responded to a series of potencies, beginning with 200C and going up to 50M over a period of a few years. With the severity of her lameness and the great concern of my client, I did not want to risk a larger aggravation from a higher potency at the start. As it was, she made slow and steady progress, and she has been limp-free for well over three years.

Remedies are tools for the vital force rather than a means to control symptoms.

This chapter has given you a real-life taste for a few different potencies, showing how a single dose can make long-lasting salutary changes. If we view remedies as tools employed by the vital force to turn the body towards the work of healing, then we will use them more advantageously. If we think of remedies as controlling the patient and his symptoms, we will be led back into the trap of symptomatic treatment. As stewards of the vital force, we optimize conditions so that health will result, rather than manipulating symptoms so that our patient looks good on the outside. Homeopathy is a different approach that requires a sense of humility, lots of patience, scholarly study, and a firm hand on our pride.

• • •

Enjoy the following cases as an illustration of the potential for homeopathy to help our animals.

The Panting Dog

Otis is an 11 year-old yellow Labrador with severe panting. Homeopathic treatment not only resolved his panting, but helped Otis regain much of the strength he had lost over the years. Unlike his elderly canine friends who looked very arthritic, moving stiffly and slowly, Otis stood out. As a 13 year-old, he was again moving at a good pace, running and playing.

The Cat With a Cold

Queenie, a young cat rescued from the town dump, had had black crusty plugs of discharge in her nose for several months. Constant cleaning didn't prevent the build-up. After her remedy she became "jet-propelled," and her nose is still clean well over a year later.

The Depressed Dog

Gal was sad and listless after losing her dog companion. She was laying around, not eating. She spent all her time alone upstairs, looking out the window, as if waiting for her friend to come home. Gal acted like an old dog, yet she was only two years old. She had also developed a smelly ear infection that was resistant to treatment. After her remedy she returned to her happy, playful, interactive self, and her ears cleared, too.

• • •

Chapter 7 References

1. Hahnemann S. *Organon of Medicine, Sixth Edition*. Künzli J, Naudé A, and Pendleton P, eds. Blaine, WA: Cooper Publishing;1982: 202.
2. *Ibid.*
3. Mish FC, Morse JM, Gilman EW, *et al.*, eds. *Merriam Webster's Collegiate Dictionary*. Springfield, MA: Merriam-Webster, Inc.; 1996: 1121.
4. *Ibid.* 1.
5. *Ibid.*, p. 202-203.
6. Close S. *The Genuis of Homoeopathy.* New Delhi, India: B. Jain Publishers;1997: 189.
7. *Ibid.*, p. 192.

8. *Ibid.* 3, p. 1187.
9. *Ibid.* 6, p. 194.
10. Winston J. *The Faces of Homœopathy an Illustrated History of the First 200 Years.* Tawa, Wellington, New Zealand: Great Auk Publishing; 1999: 54.
11. *Ibid.* 6, p. 191.
12. *Ibid.* 1, p. 127.

8 – Case Management or So I've Given the Remedy —What Happens Next?

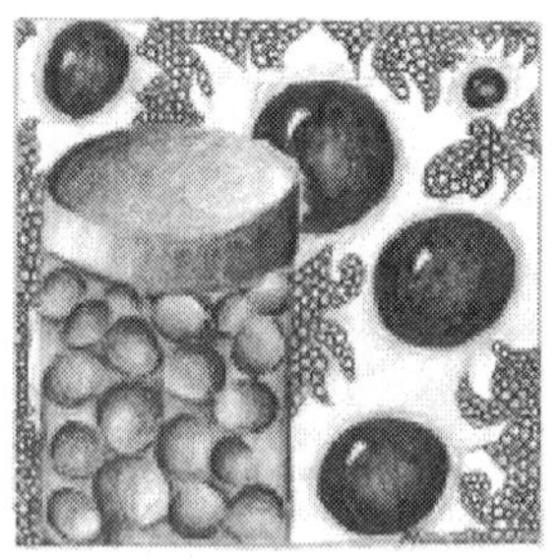

Wait as long as the case is improving.—Hahnemann, A. 246, *Organon*

After a remedy dose, patients follow their own unique paths towards health, and progress is evaluated in terms of clear and notable milestones. (For a review of the three possible responses to remedies, re-visit the chapter The Basics.) This is different from the response to allopathic medicine. With allopathy, the only real signposts are symptoms disappearing and then returning, indicating the need for a stronger dose of the palliative medicine. Over time, one symptom complex might finally disappear, and another more serious one come in its place, thus requiring a different type of palliation. The focus is quite clearly on the medication, rather than the patient.

In homeopathy, the treatment wakes up the vital force and it begins the work of healing itself. Aggravations happen, demonstrating the body's ability to rid itself of disease. Your cat or dog experiences greater energy and that long-lost brightness returns to their eyes. Toys, gathering dust in the corner, find their way back into the middle of the living room. There may be a discharge, and the appetite returns for good, wholesome foods. The mood improves, and walks, formerly cut short, become longer again. Each patient comes to life in their own way. After a period of time, symptoms of old illnesses return, which your homeopath will greet with great joy, as they are an excellent sign of true healing. The body is finally strong enough to repair those old disabilities, and greater vigor and increased enjoyment of life come hand-in-paw with such events.

Such texture and individualization were not taught to your veterinarian in medical school, because our patients were palliated and suppressed rather than given healing remedies that engage the entire body. Even blood work can't measure the progress towards health so exactly, because the details of symptom expression and response are so much more unique to the patient than red blood cell numbers and how much waste products are excreted by the kidneys or how elevated the enzymes are in the liver. Enjoy watching the stages of your animal's response as if they are a fascinating movie with an unknown plot line. Revel in the details, for each patient is following her own unique path to healing.

• • •

There is a cycle in homeopathic treatment. In the beginning, your veterinarian is connected closely to you, talking about your animal, listening carefully to your words and watching your animal companion waiting patiently (or not!) in the examination room. Then the veterinarian connects to the patient, first with an examination and then through careful study and case analysis. Homeopaths seek deep understanding of the imbalance in our patients, so we can match it with the best treatment. Next, you administer the remedy, and the focus of your veterinarian goes back onto you. When is the next appointment? What kinds of information will be needed then? What are your goals with your animal? How long will it all take?

Details are important.

A good homeopath will be as clear as possible, without making any promises. You can expect a follow-up within a few days with rapidly-progressing diseases or delicate patients, one week for sturdier stronger patients, and two weeks or more for animals with minor or slowly-progressive illnesses. Your first follow-up appointment might be longer than subsequent ones, because you hone your observational skills over time and practice. Many of us new to homeopathy don't realize that details are important. Take for example the stools, if the digestive tract is the seat of your animal's disease. You might notice not just their frequency, but color and odor, and whether the stool is difficult or easy. Your homeopath will want to know what's happened, what's changed, and by how much. Don't get out the microscope and write hourly notes, but do take notice of new things and when they happened. When did he finally start finishing his breakfast? When did she come back to the bed to sleep by your side, in her formerly favorite spot? When did he have a burst of energy? Remember Queenie, the jet-propelled cat?

During the periods between remedy doses, your homeopath will also help you address any minor complaints with gentle non-suppressive treatments. This is because the usual medications for diarrhea, itching, eye or ear conditions, for example, are suppressive by their very nature. They have been designed to stop the symptom as quickly and completely as possible. Remember in the chapter on Back to Basics how the vital force has three different responses to medicines? Suppression, palliation, and cure. We always go for the cure.

By addressing your animal's needs without the use of allopathic medications, we allow the vital force to continue unperturbed in its response to the healing remedy.

It's a process. Veterinarians and clients don't suddenly become completely comfortable in this new system. We study and learn about what it means to heal, allowing the awareness and understanding to grow slowly over time. Together we are changing a lifetime of habits. Your veterinarian will let you know what might happen in your animal, then you work together to help the process. The body is likely to respond in areas which have shown symptoms in the past. For example, a dog who used to have trouble with diarrhea is likely to have diarrhea again when reacting to the remedy. A finicky cat might have trouble with her appetite, perhaps snubbing even more foods for a time. As champions of the vital force, we learn to take careful note of what is happening, then take steps to care for the animal while they heal. We learn that ear infections can be handled with a gentle herbal rinse while waiting for the body to respond to the remedy.

We see that just cleaning out the eye discharge is sufficient to keep the patient comfortable while he is reacting to the remedy dose.

Waiting for things to get better, with clarity and forethought, is a new skill.

Follow-ups and What to Expect

"*When there is an ever-so-slight beginning of improvement, the patient will demonstrate a greater degree of comfort, increasing composure, freedom of spirit, increased courage—a kind of returning naturalness.*"
—Hahnemann, A. 253, *Organon*

Over time, we start to realize that little changes like no longer laying in the sun are definitely worth noticing and reporting. At first, the follow-ups are close together, until you are used to reporting accurately and completely, and your veterinarian's focus can go back from educating you to evaluating the patient. A follow-up physical examination is only the tip of the iceberg. Your homeopath needs much more information than that gained by an exam. When evaluating remedy reactions, your homeopath will need observations from those closest to the patient in his everyday life. How is his sleep? How does he react to the mailman now? How is she getting along with her housemates? Still having dreams? Vomiting happening less, and only a bit of liquid instead of his whole dinner? Has anything new happened that affected the household? These observations are pure gold to the homeopath, and without these he cannot help your animal. You are the key. You are your veterinarian's eyes and ears.

• • •

Here's a real-life example of an excellent follow-up report: "I've been back for a week. Just about every morning since then, [he] has had mucus in his eyes. First the left then right then left again, kind of trading off. He has major dander! Urgent poops yesterday evening. This morning the poop was very mucousy. Light spots on his nose. Red lines on his gums—not very dark though. Smell—not too bad. I really brushed him. The undercoat did not come out readily. Again lots of dander. Not too much stuff in ears. Very vocal! Movement with dreaming. Big "humfs" sounds when he lays down or moaning when he goes down. Very clingy to me. Extremely patient with [a friend's dog]. He's listening pretty well."

• • •

In the beginning, your veterinarian might choose to delineate a few key symptoms to put on the watch list. This will focus you and get you used to seeing the ebb and flow displayed by a vital force reacting to a remedy. You will begin to break out of the "the symptom is still happening" mentality, and move into the "things are changing, moving back and forth but getting less overall" mindset instead. Keep reminding yourself that remedy responses are organic, not cut-and-dried. They are individual, not one-size-fits-all. This patient is a living force who responds in fluid ways to the impression of a remedy. Remember the stuck truck? The workmen (the remedy) might shove, and the truck starts to coast. Then when the truck starts to slow down, another shove. But constant shoves are neither productive nor necessary. We are asking the vital force to wake up and respond, not setting it onto a treadmill of medicines to keep it going. To achieve this change in mind-set takes time and repetition of the principles.

"*As long as there is a marked, obviously progressing improvement during treatment, no more medicine of any kind must be given, because all the good that the medicine taken can accomplish is speeding toward its completion.*"
—Hahnemann, A. 246, *Organon*

At your follow-ups, a good homeopath will continue to avoid yes or no questions. How has the energy been? How is his thirst? How did he behave when you had guests over the holidays? Your vet will avoid specific questions which invite narrow lifeless answers that have more to do with being a compliant client than with delivering an accurate picture of the patient. You are connected with your patient and your vet is not, so when you describe a severe worrisome symptom, she wants to know what you are seeing and why it is worrisome, not yes that happened and no I didn't see that aspect of that particular symptom. Don't limit your answers to "yes" or "no."

What also helps are frequency reports of some events. For example, before the remedy he was coughing twenty times per day. How is that now? This helps determine whether the symptom is getting worse or better. It also gives you a reference point when you look back over several follow-ups. Some clients want to please their doctor, so they say "better" every time, but if asked for the actual frequency, it might become obvious that it hasn't changed that much. It's good to pin "better" down with a number from time to time. But don't focus only on the numbers. Your homeopath will also want to know how the symptom affects the patient, what time of day it's happening, how severe it is, whether it interrupts daily activities or not, and so forth. Texture is important to the homeopath.

Symptoms that bother the patient are more critical than those that don't.

Why Do I Have to Wait?

Waiting is key. After a remedy dose, waiting allows the vital force to react to the remedy. We wait and watch. If we jump in too soon with another dose, or a different remedy, then we will see only the initial reaction and we will not be allowing the curative reaction to begin. It is quite possible to palliate with a curative remedy. Just give it too often. Homeopaths seek to stimulate the vital force into healing, rather than continually medicating symptoms in order to control their expression. Infrequent dosing is best, to allow the work of the vital force free reign. Rushing with remedy doses cannot speed up the process. It only leads to disarray. This is a cardinal rule.

Old symptoms, though perhaps fearful to see, are a good sign of curative action. Let them happen.

Waiting is not the same as allowing suffering. Yes, we are just watching when the patient's symptoms begin or aggravate, but the situation is not the same as before entering homeopathic treatment. The story has changed. That ear infection that used to progress to horrible stinky pus in the past may not necessarily progress down the same road during homeopathic care. That hotspot may not get as bad as it did before the vital force was engaged. Homeopathy wakes up the vital force and then veterinarian and client must step back and let it do its work. Remember that often after a remedy the energy increases, the appetite improves, and the emotions lift? Those returning old symptoms that used to cause such suffering now occur in a newly vitalized patient. Healthier animals can endure symptoms better than they did in the past. Wait and see what might happen. Be ready with appropriate home care (discussed in the Supportive Care chapter), but allow symptoms to unfold. With proper prescribing, your animal will move past this stage and go on to greater health.

Prognosis, Or What Can I Expect From This New Medicine?

Each patient is different, even when the same disease label applies. One hyperthyroid cat may react quickly and abruptly, another may show tiny ongoing changes over a few months. One cancer patient may achieve great progress, another may only be able to slow his decline before the end. Not every patient has enough vital energy left to respond, and not every patient can be cured. But your veterinarian will use his knowledge of disease progression to evaluate your animal's prognosis. He will watch and see what happens after a remedy dose, and from this gain more information about the patient. Your veterinarian knows the singularity of each patient's disease, and how a disease label no longer comes with a one-size-fits-all life expectancy. All those estimates are turned on their heads when we confront the truth of the wonderful individuality of each patient. Prognosis is based more on the patient's vital strength rather than a disease name.

Every patient is unique. Remember how disease begins in the energetic sphere, then progresses to the level of sensation, then function, and from there to pathology? Patients with pathological changes will heal slower, if they can heal at all, due to the advanced nature of their disease. Patients with problems in multiple body systems will also take longer to show results. Young, vigorous patients will react more quickly and completely, and with more clarity, making it easier to determine the next step. Also very important to remember is that patients with guardians who communicate clearly and accurately will enable the homeopath to do their very best work.

The order of response is not always predictable. That bad symptom that brought you to homeopathy in the first place may not be the first to improve. While often the most recently-acquired symptoms are the first to resolve, this is not set in stone. Be prepared for the first response to be in a minor symptom, not necessarily the symptom most bothersome to you. This can be a frustrating aspect of homeopathic treatment. The patient decides what is resolved first—not you, not your veterinarian, and not the medicine.

Communication

Before treatment begins, your veterinarian might have you read and sign a practice disclosure statement. This simply states that they will be treating the patient with homeopathy and no other means. If in their opinion other means are necessary, then they will refer you to a specialty practice. One example of a disclosure statement, called the "Client Acceptance Form," is found in the References at the end of this book. This paper informs you and protects your veterinarian, making it clear that she is not mixing different modalities. Of course if your veterinarian does use different modalities, the client acceptance form may read differently. In all cases, clear communication is a must. Ask questions. Find out what training your veterinarian has received, and how often she uses homeopathy in her practice. If she practices other modalities, ask why, and how she chooses the modality for each particular patient.

Invoicing

No discussion of homeopathic veterinary practice would be complete without a money talk. If your veterinarian wants to practice homeopathy, she will need to pay her bills while doing it. Some homeopaths charge by time spent, similarly to lawyers. They keep careful track of minutes spent working on the cases, determine a fair hourly fee, and then invoice their clients regularly. If your homeopath does good work, then your hospital visits will decrease dramatically. Your goal, after all, is to heal your animal companion so that they don't need the veterinarian any more. Time well spent! Veterinarians may give some time away, preferring to work harder to be sure of their prescription choices. That is every practitioner's prerogative. You might see this "free" time on your invoice and be surprised by the amount of time taken for your animal. The practice of homeopathy is a time-consuming, difficult, and occasionally nerve-wracking profession. But seeing your animal blossom under the care of a good homeopath is worth every penny.

Appointment Reminders

One key to the continued progression of healing is the follow-up reminder. If your animal goes too long between treatments, progress can get bogged down, or even worse, you might be tempted to seek refuge in suppressive medications. You may see a wonderful response of the condition at first, followed by the re-emergence of a puppyhood problem. Your first instinct may be to rush to suppress this old symptom, caught up in bad memories of what happened when you last saw this symptom, and how much suffering was involved before it finally went away. Resist your impulse to grab those old medications that "worked before." Remember that medications designed for a particular symptom, not chosen based on the whole case, are suppressive. Suppressing these old symptoms could very likely cause your animal to be incurable. Contact your homeopath, tell them your fears, explain what you are seeing, and they will remind you of the vital force's healing response. Given time, these old symptoms will subside again as the patient gets stronger. If the old symptoms are uncomfortable, your veterinarian can work with you to reduce their impact while allowing the vital force to continue its healing work. Good communication with your veterinarian can head off any rash moves and settle your (very natural) feelings of desperation and fear. Don't skip your follow-ups.

Set a reminder in your calendar for those follow-up appointments. Then update your vet, even if things are going well. She cannot predict every reaction of every patient, but if old problems come up during the course of treatment, you want her prepared. If you've stayed in close touch before the flare-up, she will be ready with an action plan. Good homeopaths may even be able to warn you. Armed with their exhaustive intake notes and their close and personal knowledge of each of their patients, they can prepare you with likely scenarios. "Often old problems come back again once healing really gets going, so don't be surprised when Maxie starts having those soft stools again. Let me know right away and we'll talk about what to do next." Remember suppression, and also how the body rids itself of chronic disease (often through discharges). Remember that old problems were never really cured, only made to temporarily disappear, and that with curative treatment these old problems finally come back to be healed.

If you can't immediately reach your veterinarian, you might be moved to use another dose of the homeopathic remedy when you see symptom recurrences. Avoid this at all costs, because it is often harder to treat cases mismanaged with homeopathic remedies than cases given emergency treatment at the local veterinary hospital. If you are faced with taking your animal to the emergency hospital versus giving them a dose of remedy on your own, head to the emergency room. Do not prescribe on your own without explicit instructions from your veterinarian. Otherwise, his ability to help your animal will be severely compromised. Remember that we are dealing directly with the vital force, and many of our animals are heavily suppressed. When coming out from under suppression, unpredictable outbursts can happen. Symptoms can flare, discharges can explode, old conditions that you never wanted to see again can come back with a vengeance. The vital force must be allowed to continue its work with a trained guide at the ready. Hunker down, administer good nursing care, call your homeopath, and then wait for the storm to subside. Give it time.

Not all homeopaths are able to be at the phone 24 hours a day. This work is very time-consuming and requires absolute concentration. They will let you know how to proceed in the case of emergencies, and what to do if common troubles come up. Take notes and listen to their advice, and it will get better. Giving a dose of remedy is not like giving an aspirin—it requires serious knowledgeable study and careful patient evaluation. Good communication is key.

Diagnostics

Another aspect of case management is the use of diagnostics such as blood work, radiography, and ultrasound. These can be very helpful to augment follow-up consults and examinations. But your homeopath won't let unchanging or even worsening blood work necessarily cause her to change prescriptions which have been bringing more life to your companion. This is because blood work often lags behind real healing changes. Once sure of the prescription, your veterinarian might delay blood work longer than the allopathic practitioner. He might wait that extra month to re-check thyroid levels, for example. Remember, the prescription is determined by the patient and his symptoms. So hold on a bit before you have that blood drawn again. Diagnostics can document success, but if done too early they can also discourage and mislead client and clinician. Also, especially in feline patients, the trip to the veterinary clinic can be emotionally traumatic, setting back progress in the early weeks. This must be taken into consideration for the nervous delicate patient. If another exam is required, ask about a house call. Some veterinary practices can offer this.

The other considerations with diagnostics are expense and physical trauma. Years ago I successfully treated a bull mastiff with a malignant osteosarcoma on her front leg. (Diagnosed with a biopsy.) She was given six weeks to live. The tumor was a bony lump which only shrank slightly during homeopathic treatment over the next four years. In her case, I did not prescribe another biopsy, since that would have entailed anesthesia and a painful procedure, simply to prove a point. She was well, happy, and her lameness had disappeared. A follow-up biopsy was unwarranted. And not cheap!

• • •

A Puppy with Giardia and Chronic Diarrhea

Jake couldn't free himself of Giardia (a protozoan intestinal parasite) despite repeated courses of metronidazole (an antibiotic which targets intestinal organisms). Finally, after three months on antibiotics, his guardian turned to homeopathy. Jake not only cleared the diarrhea, but the Giardia disappeared as well.

A Cat with Inflammatory Bowel Disease

Gail, only five years old, had been on prednisone for four months for vomiting, decreased appetite, and weight loss. Her guardian, facing a lifetime of medications for her cat, wanted a better way. Homeopathy got Gail off the prednisone, stopped her vomiting, and improved her appetite. She regained her weight and now eats with gusto, even treating her housemates better than ever before.

The Dog Who Itched Herself Raw

Audrey is a young dog who chewed herself raw with regularity. She was usually treated with prednisone, but when someone suggested homeopathy, her guardian decided to give it a try. A single remedy dose stopped Audrey's itching and cleared up her skin.

9 – The Second Prescription

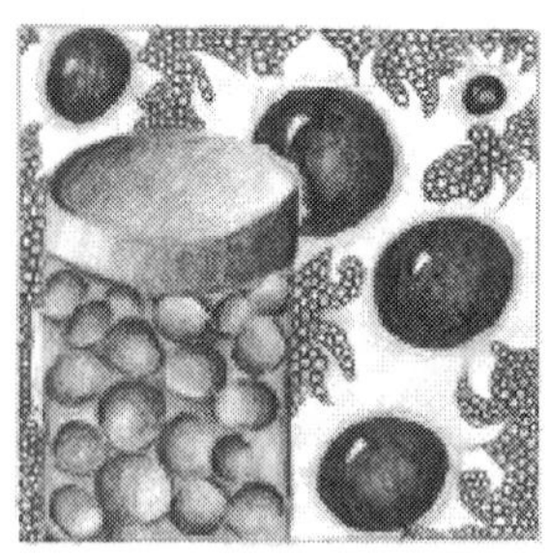

The second prescription refers to the steps taken after the first remedy has acted. Henriques puts it best: "At the second prescription stage, the patient has had the first prescription and we are waiting for the reaction of the vital force to display itself. This is the moment we've been waiting for, the moment patient and practitioner should observe the curative power of homoeopathy. We are on the edge of our seats with suspense waiting to see how close we came to matching the remedy to the symptom image totality. Within minutes in acute treatment, hours, days or weeks in chronic treatment, the patient's response to the first prescription indicates the beginning of gentle, rapid restoration of health or continued decline. If cure has begun, we glimpse the exciting possibility of the individual fulfilling full mental, emotional, and physical potential."[1]

Or to put it more succinctly, "The great challenge of the second prescription lies in confirming that the first prescription acted, understanding how and why it acted or didn't act, and deciding with confidence what to do next."[2]

Did the Remedy Act?

So what did happen? Your veterinarian will ask for a report, augmented by careful questioning. She will work from her symptom list so that nothing is missed. Even if you report no changes, she will most likely ask about each symptom. When carefully questioned, you might realize that actually some things *have* changed, other than the primary symptom that is of most concern. Then she will want to know exactly what improved and by how much, and what got worse and in what way.

So did the remedy act? If after examining each symptom you and your vet still can't be sure, then time is your friend. What happens when you wait? You hone your observational skills just a bit more, so that you are now primed to notice changes. Also, the subtle changes in your cat or dog may magnify over time and become clearer. The next follow-up may very well present that missing clarity. Don't be afraid to wait. In the meantime, you can ask for any home care regimens and dietary changes that will support the vital force of your animal without distracting from the business of healing. (See the chapter on Supportive Care.)

Waiting often brings clarity.

If the remedy did not act, and your veterinarian's assessment does not change after the second follow-up, it's time to re-examine the case. New symptoms that do not lie in the sphere of the prescription may hint at a new remedy. Or if there are no new symptoms, and the state of the patient continues unchanged, a decision has to be made. Before giving up on that remedy, your veterinarian might decide to raise the potency. Remember that not just the remedy, but the potency must also match the illness in your animal.

Generally, a good strategy is to increase the potency gradually, starting low and ending high, then returning back to low if needed, over time. Here is what Dr. Farrington, a well-respected homeopath who practiced in the early 1900's recommends: "As a rule, it is advisable to start a chronic case with the 30th or 200th. [C potencies.] There are two advantages to be gained by this procedure – the initial aggravation which sometimes follows a well chosen remedy in a higher potency is less likely to occur; and, more important still, it affords an opportunity of administering the remedy in a series of ascending potencies. Prescribers who limit themselves to the 30th, for instance, many times fail to obtain the full curative action of a remedy. The fact that the 30th or 200th has ceased to benefit the patient is not necessarily an indication that another remedy must be found. Usually improvement is re-established under the action of a higher potency of the same remedy. If this does not complete the cure and the remedy is still indicated, a still higher potency should be given. If, then, the symptoms still call for the remedy but the highest potency has exhausted its power, the clinician may return to the 200th or lower and again ascend the scale. By this method the fullest curative action of the remedy may be obtained."[3] Henriques explains, "Repeating the ascending scale works because the vital force, less burdened by symptoms, is now more open and susceptible at a deeper level to the potentized homoeopathic medicine the second time round."[4] The second time around, everything is lined up, the corners are smoothed, and the path well-lit.

Determining the Action of the Remedy

If the remedy did act, and symptoms have changed, your veterinarian's next task is to determine whether the action of the remedy was palliative, suppressive, or curative. (For a review, refer to the chapter The Basics.) If the symptoms have improved, but only at the outermost edges of the case, then the remedy may be palliative at that potency. In this situation, your veterinarian might prescribe a higher potency of the same remedy. Since superficial improvements with a palliative remedy are even shorter-lasting and more superficial when the potency is increased, this could make the situation more clear. With palliation, discharges may ease, odors may lessen, and the skin may get less inflamed, but there is no increase in vitality or overall well-being. It's time to re-take the case and give a new prescription.

Was the remedy response suppressive? Are symptoms no longer being expressed, and the patient even sicker, if only subtly? Your homeopath might decide to re-take the case, looking at his notes and questioning you again. Perhaps one symptom has become stronger, more important, and others more inconsequential. These follow-up conversations often put the finishing touch to the intake interview, given the perspective of time and more valuable information that you can now provide with your greater understanding. Your eyes may be opened in a way they had not been before, allowing you to appreciate symptoms as messengers rather than annoyances. This new clarity is of immense benefit to your homeopath as he takes a fresh look.

Was the remedy curative? Now what? Give it again and again, right? Quickly, so that the patient can be well? No! Remember that the process of cure is organic, not mechanical. You cannot simply push harder to force the disease to go away quicker. It is a balancing, a tuning, freeing the vital force from chronic disease so that it can finally breathe deeply and correct its unhealthy state. This takes time and respect for the natural timetable of each patient. Your homeopath's job is to determine when the next push is needed. So for the first follow-up, during a curative action, the main focus is to set the time for the next appointment.

As long as improvement continues, no medicine is required.

Once improvement ceases, your vet will often counsel you to wait longer. This is because vital interior work could still be happening, invisible from the outside. We are not able to access the inner thoughts and feelings of our patients, so as veterinary practitioners, we must give extra leeway to allow healing to continue without disturbance. Keep in close touch, but wait until there is a decline. Once this happens, the vital force is clearly calling for more medicine.

If the patient is getting well but some new symptoms appear, your vet will re-visit your animal's timeline. Are these forgotten historical symptoms? This is a very good sign that healing is taking place and old issues are being resolved. This is also the hardest time to wait and not medicate (for both practitioner and client). Often these old symptoms were associated with great discomfort, and you may (understandably) be quite dismayed at their re-occurrence. However, the situation is not the same as it was in the past. Your animal is healthier, and engaged in the business of healing, rather than fighting suppression. These old symptoms will most likely pass on their own, given time. Ask your veterinarian about home care therapies that will support and nurture, rather than suppress. Now your animal is stronger, so the suffering will not be intense like it was when the symptom was new. Keep in close touch with your vet during this difficult time. Ask questions when you have them. Allow time and space for healing.

If the symptoms coming up are totally new, either the remedy is not a complete match but can still be partially helpful, or the remedy needs to be changed. It is also possible, for animals with multiple guardians, that the symptom occurred in another household and was never mentioned. Wait for things to settle down. Your vet will not change remedies unless the symptoms become persistent. Another sign that the remedy is wrong is that these new symptoms become more obvious and distressing after the second dose of remedy. But if this doesn't happen, a minor new symptom that resolves on its own is not cause for concern or a reason to change prescriptions. The treatment has brought out remedy symptoms, but in this case they do not go deep into the case, being minor and short-lived. The remedy is still a good match.

Timing: Important to Get it Right

Timing is an under-appreciated issue. This is because we all came from the allopathic mode, where medicine is only appreciated for its action on the most bothersome symptoms. By contrast, with homeopathic remedies, we are striving to involve the vital force. This takes time. Palliation and suppression are actions taken upon the vital force by medicines. Cure, on the other hand, is action *initiated* by the remedy but *taken up and maintained* by the vital force. The medicine is no longer in charge. We, who administer the medicine, are no longer in charge. So when you are waiting for the remedy action to finish, how does your veterinarian decide when another dose of medicine is needed? When is it too early to dose? When should you wait? Here are some guidelines to read over and digest:

• • •

When is another dose of medicine needed?

Symptoms have calmed down for awhile, then have started intensifying again.
Symptoms have been unchanging and stable for a few weeks to a month.
New symptoms appear and stay, and they match the remedy.
The patient appears to be sicker in himself again, and is not rallying.

When is another dose NOT necessarily indicated?

When you run out of doses in the remedy bottle or packet.
When the patient's symptoms flare up, but he is still well in himself.
When symptoms reappear, but at a lesser intensity than before treatment began.

When nothing seems to be changing.
When new symptoms appear and don't bother the patient unduly.
When the patient isn't getting well fast enough.
When you want to speed things up in general.
When you are about to take a vacation and want everything to be fine when you are away.
When you don't know what else to do.

. . .

Once you and your homeopath have determined that the remedy is no longer acting, even at a higher potency, or that new and persistent symptoms have appeared, then it is time for a decision. The patient needs more help, but is the same remedy indicated, just at a higher potency? Or is it time to change remedies?

When is a change of remedy indicated?

	repeat current remedy	new prescription needed
patient healthier overall	X	
lengthy prior amelioration	X	
similar or milder symptom intensity	X	
(still) no amelioration of symptoms		X
very short amelioration of symptoms		X
no overall improvement		X
feeling worse overall		X
symptoms are stronger in intensity		X
new symptom(s) not fitting prescription		X

. . .

New Symptoms

When a new symptom appears, don't panic. First your homeopath will determine whether the rubric which comes closest to this new symptom contains the patient's remedy. If so, then there is no need to change the remedy, because the symptom still corresponds to the current prescription. For further confirmation, your vet will check the materia medica for that remedy, to see if the new symptom is described well in the provings. Often this provides further confirmation of the remedy. Finally, he will examine the rest of the case to determine whether the remedy action up to this point appears curative. If it is, then he will urge you to wait out this new symptom, and he will not change the remedy. Our patients come with complex reactions that don't always exactly follow the formula of cure. Sometimes the remedy outline is just a bit different than the patient's disease, so the extra areas not matching the disease's outline stir up new symptoms. This does not mean the remedy is unsuitable. Your homeopath will examine his case notes carefully before making any decision. As Kent writes, "The medicine that has partly cured the case can often finish it, and that medicine should not be changed until there are good reasons for changing it."[5]

If, however, your vet determines that the new symptom does not fit the current remedy, and it persists and becomes a bother to the patient, do not despair. Re-taking the case is not a failure, and this time it will be easier because of your experience with the process and your veterinarian's extensive notes.

. . .

Here's a case of aggression to illustrate the need for a change of remedy. Hedrick is a male short-haired domestic cat:

Hedrick's timeline:

2004	year of birth; early vaccines; never sociable; "always underfoot and always into something;" was neutered during his first year
2006	moved across the country
1/08	bit the veterinarian during a wellness check
7/15/08	husband returned to work; Hedrick began attacking other cats
9/2/08	diarrhea after a new food
9/27/08	crying, irritable, attacks guests
10/2/08	urinating excessive amounts; treated with homeopathy, then onset of abdominal gas
12/22/08	nasty

• • •

Hedrick's symptoms:

short fuse, flares in a second
    worse for attention
    worse for contradiction
    worse in the late afternoon
    better for routines
walks and cries when the guardian leaves
desires sunlight
diarrhea like brown water, worse with a change of diet
    gas worse after eating, "like trash left too long"
    belches after eating
mounting of stuffed animals or blankets (sexual posturing)
frequent urination
    straining, worse after urinating
    sour urine with a pinkish tint

• • •

Progress of Hedrick's case (see the chapter Case Analysis for a review of repertorization):

1/23/09 sepia 200C	follow-up in three weeks
2/20/09	subtle amelioration two weeks after the prescription; but last two weeks actually worse; really nasty when client was boxing things up
3/2/09	still bats at other cats if prevented from doing what he wants to do; hissed at a guest; no diarrhea or gas

• • •

Did the remedy act? First Hedrick was improved, then he was clearly worse. These changes occurred on the mental and emotional planes. This could be due to the remedy. However, it is possible that this is his normal pattern, simply exacerbated by the activities associated with packing up for moving the household. I decided to wait longer.

• • •

3/16/09	(7 ½ weeks after the sepia) aggression escalating; "never seen him worse, really in a mood;" confrontational; bit three times when guardian tried to clean the counter; growled and charged when ignored; almost daily aggression now

• • •

Clearly, Hedrick is getting worse. The remedy dose has stopped helping, and now he is needing another dose. To give a slightly higher potency, I had the client dissolve a few pellets of the 200C in water and stir it vigorously for 30 seconds before dosing him with ¼ teaspoon. This is called plussing.

Since the improvement on 2/20/09 was very subtle rather than dramatic, and also since Hedrick is a young vital cat, it is possible that the remedy potency was too low. So it is definitely worth trying again, plussed.

• • •

3/16/09	sepia 200C, plussed
3/30/09	walking around purring the day after the prescription; "humping (sexual posturing);" playing with the other cats "in a way I haven't seen in awhile;" one curled up beside him (this is brand new, never happened before); but then he bit the client and broke the skin (this is new); aggression is now once or twice daily

• • •

Repeating the remedy brought clarity. There was a dramatic change, telling us that the remedy acted. The up and down swings are clearly from the treatment, not just Hedrick's normal mood changes. So what was the remedy action? With two doses of sepia over ten weeks of treatment, how has Hedrick's disease changed? He is even more aggressive to guests and other cats, and dramatically worse towards the client. This aggression now occurs once or twice a day, rather than occasionally. His attacks are more serious, at times even breaking the skin, which is new. Even ignoring him does not avoid an attack. His sexual activity was not even mentioned at the intake interview, but now it is frequent. His gas and diarrhea, old symptoms, have not recurred.

Hedrick is clearly worse, with stronger, more serious, and more easily provoked attacks. The remedy causes a brief improvement, followed by a worsening on the mental and emotional levels. Physically, his outlets, in the form of diarrhea and gas, are quiet. This is the classic picture of palliation. Time to re-work the case, using my new understanding of his modalities (aggravation even when ignored) and another added symptom (sexual activity) to the mix. After working the case again, as described in previous chapters, I settled on phosphorus.

• • •

4/6/09 phosph 200C	
4/19	more easily called off; back to sleeping in bed with the client (this is a new event since the move in 2006); some days no aggression at all; "the intensity is lower"

• • •

This response is good, but less dramatic than after the sepia. This is another hint that sepia was palliative, and the response to phosphorus potentially curative. Palliative reactions can be very dramatic, yet short-lasting. This response is more subtle, and continues to evolve. Hedrick is still aggressive, but less so and less often. He has relaxed back to his former cuddly habits of sleeping with the client at night, a habit that was lost along with the stress of the move. This shows emotional improvement in two different arenas. This response is definitely worth waiting on, to see how far it will go and how much more he will change before requiring any more assistance. So here are some highlights from the next few months. During this time, Hedrick did not receive any additional remedy doses:

• • •

4/22/09	rubbing and purring (a completely new behavior)
4/25/09	"evil twin is back"
4/27/09	lots of guests in the house; stressed, "but aggression is less intense on this remedy"
5/14/09	no reaction to guest; client "thrilled"
6/1/09	"good days and less than good ones;" rubbed guest's leg; hissed, spit, and swiped at the catsitter

. . .

See how the new behavior of rubbing and purring is happening in new situations? Hedrick is relaxing. This is a very good sign that the remedy is acting deeply. Also, his response goes up and down. This roller-coaster ride is common in the early weeks of the curative remedy. Finally, his behavior seems to decline and worsen, at which point he was given a plussed dose of the same remedy that acted so well many weeks ago.

. . .

6/26/09 phosph 200C, plussed	(two months three weeks since the last dose)
8/09	able to be brushed (hasn't happened in years); then "no more Mr. Nice Guy!" sexual activity has returned; emotionally worse for more than three consecutive days

. . .

At this point, I checked in the repertory for a rubric matching his sexual behavior. As a neutered male, sexual activity is not normal, so it would be considered increased in Hedrick. The rubric Genitalia; sex; increased desire, fits. Phosphorus, Hedrick's remedy, is present in this rubric. In the materia medica, phosphorus reads, "Satyriasis; lascivious...sexual mania; extreme irresistible desire for coition...."[6] This fits sexual behavior in a neutered male. So with this confirmation that phosphorus still fits the case, together with a clear worsening, it's time to repeat, at a higher potency.

. . .

8/20/09 phosph 1M	(seven weeks since the last dose)
9/20	occasional sexual activity (improved); no gas or diarrhea;

	sleeping in bed 50% of the time; testiness less often (kitchen counter confrontations only 25% of the time instead of every time); may cry if left alone; tolerates brushing; growling mostly only for visitors; overall improved emotionally

• • •

His improvements have held in that he tolerates brushing and his sexual activity has lessened, and his aggression towards the client is ameliorated. Worth waiting on!

• • •

11/5/09 phosph 1M plussed	(2 ½ months since the last dose) given after backsliding again
11/27/09	"this dosing had little effect;" sexual activity; pinning other cats; irritable and aggressive most of the time with visitors; nasty on the counter

• • •

Increasing the potency by plussing was not enough. Not much changed, and now his aggression is worsening. Time to increase the potency.

• • •

12/13/09 phosph 10M	
12/23/09	"a slight shift;" lays on client (unusual for him); "just can't get enough cuddles;" coming to bed again; still mounting; appetite OK

• • •

This is a good time to step back and see what phosphorus has accomplished in Hedrick's case. After eight months and five doses, he is still sexually active, and his appetite is generally good (notice how his appetite was not brought up at the intake but seems to be a concern now, so I will add it to my symptom list for future reference). Hedrick now likes attention, but he still displays major aggression with guests. He is constantly underfoot (this may just be his personality, not an expression of disease, as it hasn't changed at all with his other remedy reactions), and his behavioral flare-ups are now daily. Again we reach another crossroads, when the helpful remedy stops helping, even at a higher potency. Some things are better, in that he is now cuddly and the aggression is directed more outside the family, but overall he is not well. He is still an aggressive unhappy cat in certain situations.

Another sign of non-curative action is that Hedrick's past symptoms of diarrhea and gas never returned. So I studied his case again, then re-repertorized to see if there was a better remedy. Sulfur was a good match.

• • •

2/5/10 sulfur 30C	
3/30/10	"no effect;" now sleeping under the blankets
4/16/10	vomiting episodes over three days
5/10/10	a general calming, sense of well-being, eating well, no counter confrontations

• • •

Overall things are much better, though it was a very slow reaction to the 30C. Now, three months after the dose, there are only a few little flare-ups, there is little response to guests, Hedrick is eating well, and he doesn't even confront the client when she is cleaning the counter!

When Hedrick ramped up again in August 2010, he received sulfur 200C. This was six months after the 30C dose. Three days after the remedy he was "extremely agitated;" since then his mood "improved a little," he has had moderate reactions to guests, and he is no longer nasty with the client. Over the next 13 months, he became less clingy, he was "not too much of a pest," and during one whole week he did not confront the catsitters! His counter run-ins stopped, and his aggression overall came to an end. What a happy result! It took time and occasional re-working, but overall he is in a far better place and more able to enjoy life without emotional turmoils. Without any return of old symptoms, I can't be sure that he is truly cured, but his life has improved dramatically and the whole family is much happier.

• • •

References Chapter 9

1. Henriques N. Crossroads to Cure: *The Homoeopath's Guide to Second Prescription*. St. Helena, CA: Totality Press; 1998: 23-24.
2. *Ibid.*, p. 25-26.
3. Farrington H. *Homoeopathy and Homoeopathic Prescribing.* New Delhi, India: B. Jain Publishers; 2001: 236.
4. *Ibid.* 1, p. 67.
5. Kent J. *Lectures on Homeopathic Philosophy*. Berkeley, CA: North Atlantic Books; 1979: 235.
6. Hering C. *The Guiding Symptoms of Our Materia Medica*. Vol. 8. Paharganj, New Delhi, India: B. Jain Publishers;1995: 353.

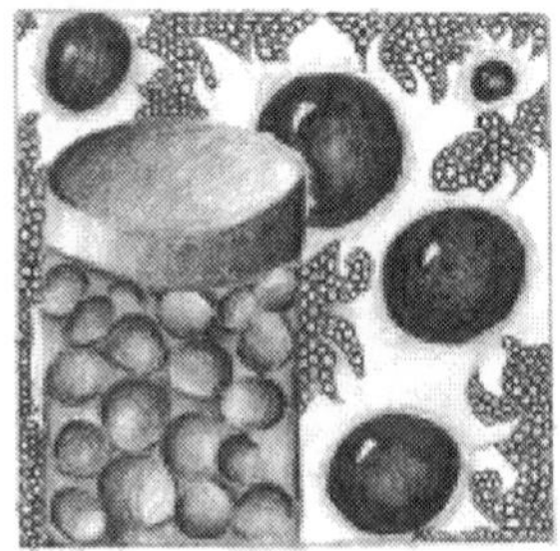

10 – Supportive Care or How to Keep That Healing Remedy Response Going

The hard work is done. We are watching and waiting to see how the healing unfolds. During this time, I'll often educate my clients about other ways to support and strengthen their companion. Now is the time to avoid any negative influences that might take away from the job of healing. One pervasive practice that must be curtailed or even eliminated in order to protect the patient is vaccination. While I cannot legally advise against the rabies vaccination, as it is required by law in many countries, the other vaccines can often be severely limited without compromising the safety of your animal.

Why limit vaccines? Because they interfere with the patient's response to homeopathic treatment (or any treatment). The vital force responds as a unit, and if the immune system is asked to react to injected foreign materials, it will not be able to respond to the remedy as well. Furthermore, repeated immune stimulation may be linked to the development of auto-immune conditions. Vaccinosis is a common chronic disease in animals, triggered by vaccines. It is passed from generation to generation, and is implicated in many conditions, such as skin allergies, epilepsy, thyroid disease, chronic hepatitis, kidney disease, cystitis, asthma, autoimmune hemolytic anemia, and even mental confusion. One excellent article discussing this topic can be found on Dr. Charles Loops' web page, at http://www.charlesloopsdvm.com/articles/vaccinosis.

Are Vaccines Safe?

Vaccines are meant to prepare the immune system for an encounter with an infectious agent. A weakened form of the virus or bacteria (or its toxins) is injected through the skin, along with chemicals designed to stimulate the immune system. Theoretically, the immune system then responds more quickly and effectively when exposed to this same infectious agent in the future. This artificial immunity mimics the natural immunity acquired through infection, without the consequences of actually getting sick. However, artificial immunity may not last as long, and this protection is not without risks.

Most infectious agents enter through the mucous membranes such as the mouth, nose, or eyes, where the immune system's cells are lined up, ready for action. When thus approached, the immune system's reaction is coordinated perfectly, the infection is controlled and moderated, and the patient acquires (in many cases) lifelong immunity. This is how it's supposed to work. But when the infectious agent is injected underneath the skin or into muscle tissue, the body's reaction is blunted, since the typical front line immune cells are not present in the same amounts. Imagine an army battalion air-lifted behind enemy lines. The checkpoints designed to process information and react to the invading virus are bypassed.

In addition, when the exposure is to a *modified* form of the infectious agent, combined with chemicals designed to artificially stimulate the immune system, the body's reactions are distorted further. Vaccination is not a natural process, but an artificially-induced manipulation of nature's protective reaction to infection. This is a recipe for auto-immune dysfunction.

These immune-stimulating chemicals are often toxic materials that we naturally avoid in other areas of our lives, such as thimerosal (a mercury derivative), anti-fungals such as benzethonium chloride, antibiotics, and tissue fixatives such as formaldehyde.[1] In addition to toxic chemicals, contaminants have historically been discovered in cell cultures used to make the vaccines, which are often grown on cells originating from other species. For example, SV40 (a virus that causes cancer in animals) has been discovered in the human polio vaccine. [2]

How Can I Protect My Animal?—Guidelines for Reducing the Impact of Vaccines

Nothing can keep your animals completely safe. There are no guarantees in the world of health care. However, aside from avoiding vaccines entirely (which many of my clients have decided to do), there are steps you can take to minimize the risk from chemical contaminants and artificial stimulation of the immune system. If possible, avoid vaccines entirely during the early stages of working with your homeopathic veterinarian. Then, if and when you decide to vaccinate, prepare your veterinarian ahead of time. Ask for only one vaccine to be given at a time, so that the animal can recover in between each injection. Also, give the vaccines at increased intervals, rather than yearly. You can also ask for a titer test (a blood test) instead of the vaccine. This measures the amount of antibody present in the patient. While not proof of immunity, a high titer is an indication that the previously-administered vaccine has done all it could do and that another injection is not needed at this time.

Also consider vaccinating only young animals, as is the general practice in human medicine. Two doses of the distemper and parvo vaccines will protect the puppy or kitten for a lifetime, according to Dr. Ronald Schultz, a pioneer in the field of veterinary vaccines. Some experts recommend the killed virus vaccine over the modified live, but this is controversial, since the killed vaccine may contain higher amounts of chemical immune-system stimulants.

You may decide to give some vaccines and not others. Many regular veterinary practices are beginning to recommend only "core" vaccines, offering the other ones only to certain "higher risk" populations. While you must talk to your local veterinarian and do your own research, I recommend avoiding the following vaccines entirely. They are either ineffective, fraught with side effects, or the disease itself is mild and can be treated with homeopathy:

• • •

Canine Vaccines to Avoid

kennel cough (Bordetella)
parainfluenza
corona
Lyme
canine hepatitis
leptospirosis

Feline Vaccines to Avoid

FIP
FeLV
chlamydia
ringworm

• • •

If you are considering reducing vaccines, and giving only the most effective long-lasting vaccines which protect against serious illnesses, then consider distemper and parvo in dogs, and panleukopenia in cats (cat distemper). Rabies is required by law. For equine vaccines, research which infectious illnesses have been a problem in your area before vaccinating. Find out if the vaccines can be spread out instead of being given yearly or every six months. Find out which vaccines are more prone to side effects. Also research the disease itself: is it serious? Can your homeopath treat it with remedies?

Ask questions. Do the research. Question the reasoning traditionally given for vaccinating your animals every year, throughout their lifetimes. Learn how the immune system is artificially stimulated to produce a response in the absence of a threat. Consider how this stimulation might predispose your animal to auto-immune conditions. Read the available literature (some suggestions included in the Reference section of this book) on vaccination and its attendant risks. Be an educated advocate for your animal.

Diet

The second way you can protect your animal and maximize the benefit gained from their homeopathic treatment is through diet and nutrition. I heartily recommend feeding a raw home-prepared diet as much as possible. Not everyone can do this, whether due to difficulties in procuring and preparing the meal at home, or frequent travel, or the lack of kitchen facilities, but any steps taken towards this ideal will be of help. If making it yourself is not an option, there are frozen raw diets available for dogs and cats, as well as mixes that can be added to kibble or canned food to raise the level of nutrition. Raw-fed animals have more energy, a brighter sparkle to their eyes, and a full, lush coat. They are more resistant to digestive difficulties, less prone to allergies, and best of all, their stools degrade faster! (Commercially-fed dogs have preservatives in their stool, which causes it to stay intact on the lawn far longer.)

What is a Raw Home-Prepared Diet?

This consists of fresh organic meat and a source of calcium, with added vitamins and minerals. There are several books on the market (see the reference section) to guide you in this most inexpensive way of feeding your dog or cat. Once you begin researching the ingredients in commercial food, you will discover everything that you will avoid by preparing meals yourself, at home. Commercial food is often made from by-products from the slaughterhouse industry, including chicken feet and heads, which don't have a lot of available nutrition. Diseased meat may also be included, such as abscesses, tumors, or bruised meat. With non-organic sources, the meat often contains hormones, antibiotic residues, and pesticides, as well as those pervasive chemical preservatives which ensure a long shelf life. Artificial colors and flavors top off the list.

Aside from the ingredients, the processing of dog or cat food is problematic. In order to achieve a long shelf life, the ingredients are subject to high temperatures (300 – 350 degrees) and pressures. This breaks down the constituent amino acids, destroys natural nutrients and enzymes, eliminates any vital energy, and combines the ingredients into toxic indigestible chemicals. We don't feed our children or ourselves solely from cans or bags. Why should we feed our animals this way?

One last recommendation for you before you begin to navigate on your own: Dry food and cats do not mix. Domestic cats are descended from desert animals, and as such they obtain most of their water from the food they eat. They do not have a strong thirst drive. When fed dry food (a dehydrated product), they end up chronically dehydrated, leaving them susceptible to kidney disease as they age. All the more reason to feed raw!

Supportive Care

When you are changing your relationship to symptoms, it helps to have some first-aid home care at the ready. Not everybody is able to stand by while their beloved animal expresses symptoms, even if it is during the course towards cure. You can prepare ahead of time, knowing what symptoms your animal has struggled with in the past. If ear infections have plagued your dog, stock up with some gentle soothing remedial treatments. If hotspots have been a concern, look up some natural treatments from the following section and have them at the ready. Vomiting cat? Have slippery elm at the ready. The aggravated symptoms won't last forever. These uncomfortable conditions will ease over time and eventually go away. Previously an unheard-of goal! Here are some suggestions to provide short-term relief without suppression. *Always check with your veterinarian before administering any treatment*. My sources are *The New Natural Cat* by Anitra Frazier, *Natural Health for Dogs & Cats* by Susan and Richard Pitcairn, DVM, and handouts by Christina Chambreau, DVM.

• • •

Home Remedies

Itching: calendula lotion, Rescue Remedy (diluted in water and sprayed on); tea tree oil (diluted and sprayed on—dogs only); goldenseal root compress for hotspots (2 tsp of the tincture per pint of water); Fels naphtha soap for hotspots (let it dry on the hotspot); vitamin E oil; aloe vera gel; oatmeal poultice; Aveeno oatmeal soap bath; witch hazel; vinegar or milk bath; Epsom salts or baking soda bath; dilute p'au d'arco (tincture found in herb stores); fasting for two days; clipping the fur short

• • •

Internal supplements to reduce itching: brewer's yeast or primary nutritional yeast (1 tsp to 3 TB, depending upon the size of your animal); garlic (1-5 cloves a day, but don't use long-term as it can be toxic); cod liver oil (contains vitamins A and D—1/8 to 1 tsp); safflower or corn oil for dogs (1 tsp to 2 TB per day); olive oil for cats (¾ tsp per day); vitamin E (30-50 I.U. per day for cats, 50-400 I.U. per day for dogs or 20-40 minim capsules of wheat germ oil per day for both); zinc (may only benefit Malamutes and Huskies—10 mg per day); lecithin (1/3 to 2/3 tsp per day); selenium (50 µg per day for dogs); Derm Caps or Opticoat II (get from veterinarians); cumin or coriander in food

• • •

Fleas: The best defense is a very healthy animal. PetGuard Yeast and Garlic Powder, given throughout the year, can reduce your cat or dog's attractiveness to fleas.
(http://www.petguard.com/dog-products/supplements/yeast-and-garlic).

Some non-chemical flea repellents include fresh lemon juice; dilute citronella or pennyroyal oil (dogs only); and Avon's Skin So Soft. Daily flea combing is a must. Also investigate the natural products available in pet stores. If the fleas are inside, treat the house with diatomaceous earth (found in feed stores) and daily vacuuming (empty the vacuum bag daily). A bowl of soapy water with a lamp shining on it may also attract and kill fleas.

• • •

Additional supplements for general health (especially if you are feeding processed foods): Standard Process whole food supplements (have to be ordered by your veterinarian — https://www.standardprocess.com/Veterinary-Formulas#.Vehah3Xd-iu); vitamin C (sodium ascorbate powder) for any chronic disease, or during stress (500-2,000 mg per day, depending upon the size of your dog or cat); B vitamins (½ of a crushed 10 mg B-complex pill per day for cats); bone meal, a source of calcium (use human quality only—1/3 tsp per day for cats, 1 tsp to 1½ TB per day for dogs); Prozyme (enzyme supplement that helps animals digest foods that have been depleted of their natural enzymes by processing—get from veterinarians); Anitra's Vita-Mineral Mix (ready-made supplement for dogs and cats, containing B vitamins, calcium, phosphorus, magnesium, iron, manganese, methionine, and taurine, found at PetGuard's website at http://www.petguard.com/cat-products/supplements)

• • •

Digestive Upsets: activated charcoal for distress from eating garbage or toxic materials; Kaopectate for diarrhea (1 tsp to 1TB depending upon size), repeat every 4 hours as needed; slippery elm capsules for diarrhea and vomiting (boil 1 slightly rounded tsp powder in 1 cup cold water while stirring constantly, then simmer and stir for 2-3 minutes, cool, give ½ tsp to cats and 1 tsp—4 TB to dogs, depending upon size, four times a day)

• • •

Eye Irritation: cod liver oil drops into eyes; eyebright herb (euphrasia) (boil 3 tsp in 1 cup of water, steep 3 minutes, cool to room temperature and drop in eye three times a day); calendula non-alcoholic tincture, 5 drops per ½ cup of saline (1/8 tsp salt per ½ cup water); other tinctures that can be useful at the above strength are chamomile, goldenseal, and echinacea

• • •

Wounds: calendula, prepared as under Eye Irritation but use 10 drops per ounce of saline (note: do not use on punctures, as they heal over too fast and may form abscesses); Vitamin E capsules; calendula ointment; aloe vera plant juice for use on superficial scrapes, burns, hotspots, and wounds; goldenseal powder or salve for use on minor infected wounds or animal bites to draw out the infections; tea bags (caffeinated) when wet and placed on a hotspot may relieve the redness and heat

• • •

General emergencies, shock, emotional distress: Rescue Remedy—put two to three drops in water bowl and fill with water (also have plain water available); other Bach flower remedies for emotional upsets

• • •

With emergencies such as uncontrolled bleeding or difficulty breathing, head to your nearest veterinary hospital. Don't try to handle emergencies on your own. In some cases, the proper homeopathic remedy will alleviate severe symptoms, but do not wait at home....if you are sure of the remedy, give it *on the way to* the veterinary hospital.

• • •

These supportive measures can help you soothe and comfort your animal when they are experiencing the return of old symptoms. They can also be used in aged animals who may be nearing the end of their lifetimes. Some patients come to me when everything else has been tried and they are still sick. Often these animals have no energy left to respond to treatment. The best we can do is to ease their final days.

What Happens at the End of Life? Terminal Patients

This special scenario demands the same individualized attention we have practiced for all the prior cases in this book. What makes the end of life even more potentially confusing and complicated is the availability of euthanasia for our animal patients. Euthanasia offers a sanctioned way to schedule the "end of suffering," for both the animal and the person who loves them. When the "quality of life" is deemed to be below a certain accepted level, our society considers it desirable to end that life with an injection.

Seriously ill animals look, act, and feel differently than those in comfortable old age, and this difference is often labeled as suffering. The animal (non-human or human) approaching the end of life may first lose their appetite, often appearing nauseous when offered food, as shown by squinting, turning their head away, licking their lips, and even sometimes gagging and retching. This complete lack of appetite can very distressing to the client. It is seen as "giving up," drawing away. As loving caretakers, we may feel desperate, hurt, and even insulted until we come to accept that this is the beginning of a decline, leading inexorably to a final parting. At this point, many clients will choose to force-feed, some even having a tube surgically placed into the animal's stomach. This will definitely prolong life, and may be the best choice in young animals with a treatable disease that is not responding to homeopathic care. It can buy time. But in an aged animal who no longer has the desire for food, forcing it on their bodies will add to the suffering.

After losing their appetite, terminally ill animals will lose weight and become weak, often also losing their thirst drive. Human patients in hospices describe dehydration as being more comfortable than artificial hydration, once they no longer desire to drink. This is when the physical changes become quite obvious, such as progressive emaciation with muscle loss and weakness. Coincidentally, animals often will find a quiet out-of-the-way place to rest at this time. Their needs become very small, as they only rarely have to urinate or defecate, and they have much more time to rest, sleep, and dream. Once drinking stops, the end is no more than a few days away.

All during this process, homeopathic remedies can ease most discomforts that arise, such as nausea, restlessness, anxiety, or distressing confusion. Stay in close touch with your homeopath, as she can suggest interventions if these are warranted, and ensure that your animal does not suffer during this final time of their life. Though I have only rarely found the need for remedies in patients undergoing the dying process, consider having the following on hand to alleviate possible discomfort or distress. [Source: personal experience and Hering's *Materia Medica*.]

• • •

apis: The patient may be delirious, or semi-conscious with screaming or shrieking. They are worse from heat or even touch. There may be hot, reddish-blue swelling, and the symptoms come on with great rapidity and violence. Symptoms tend to be right-sided. Cold applications relieve. One side of the body is twitching while the other is motionless, and there is great weakness.

arsenicum: The patient is very restless, unable to settle down and sleep. Anxiety predominates, with the desire for company as displayed by clinging to the client, or if unable to rise, crying when left alone. All symptoms get worse after midnight, and the fear can suddenly peak at times, especially during the night. There may be vomiting and diarrhea, and the stool is quite offensive. The patient is thirsty but only takes small amounts at a time, which may then be vomited. There is great weakness and emaciation.

carbo-veg: Stupor and collapse, or confusion. Shuddering anxiety, easily frightened. Head painfully sensitive to pressure, eyes dull and lusterless. Hemorrhage from eyes, nose, or anus. Mouth and breath cold. Frequent empty eructations (burps). Nausea caused by eating or by the heat of the sun. Vomiting of blood. Abdominal distress with great accumulation of flatus making the stomach tense and full. Loud rumbling, with great quantities of hot moist offensive flatus. Shortness of breath with desire to be fanned. Weary after the least exertion.

opium: The patient is confused, if not completely unconscious. Glassy eyes with stupor. Flatulent colic and intestinal spasms with great pain. Involuntary stool, especially after a fright. Starting at the least noise. Twitching. Cold rigid extremities. Dry mucous membranes but hot damp skin.

veratrum album: The patient has sunken eyes and may be delirious with violent outbursts and striking out. They may faint from fright or from the least exertion, and they cannot bear to be left alone. Vomiting and purging, or constipation with large hard stools. There is great prostration with thirst, and a rapid sinking of the vital force. Convulsions. They are very chilly, and may have blue-tinged skin.

• • •

It is possible to have a peaceful death at home without machines. Some of the most poignant experiences in my practice have been during the last hours of a patient's life. The common thread to these experiences is the close connection between the dying animal and their guardian. When the time is near, the patient often sleeps for many hours a day. They may wake only occasionally, sometimes looking for company, but not always. They may prefer to be held, but more commonly prefer a soft warm area away from the business of the household. They may have no thirst or appetite (though do offer food and water occasionally just to be sure). Their bodies seem to shrink and close in upon themselves. It is not easy for the patient's loved ones, but if they have accepted that the end is near, the very real spiritual connection to their animal often deepens during these last days. Even though at the end the earthly tie is broken, something intangible is shared during the gentle peaceful passing of a loved one's life.

Euthanasia

Before I came to homeopathy, I performed many euthanasias, and found overwhelmingly that the relief of suffering had more to do with the clients than with their animal. This could be because my options, as their veterinarian, for relieving suffering, were limited in the allopathic model, mostly consisting of pain killers which are heavy with mind-numbing side effects. So when faced with the choice of an anxious restless possibly painful animal or a semi-comatose drugged body in the corner, what compassionate soul would not chose to end their beloved's life? Our animals are not burdened with a prefabricated image of what makes a "good death." They just know what is there, what is happening now, and what they are feeling in the moment. If we can keep them comfortable, then we don't have to worry about a good death. Be with them and tend to their needs, just as you have for their whole lives.

Terminal patients have different needs than chronically ill patients. Dying patients ask only for a soft warm place to sleep, rarely an offer of a drink or a bite to eat, sometimes company, and gentle respectful attention to bodily hygiene. Some of us might prefer to keep our dying animal at home, comforting them with remedies and home care, while others caretakers might panic and suffer terribly. You must do what feels right for you, and what you know is best for your animal. Close communication with your veterinarian, again, is a must. Revisit this question often, what do you want to do if....? Be prepared with remedies for the dying process, and don't hesitate to bring your animal into the hospital if that is what seems best. Dying is as unique as birthing, maybe more so, and can be honored as a normal process at the end of a long life. You might find, as I did, that patients treated with homeopathy go through the dying process more rapidly and more gently than patients suppressed throughout their lives.

• • •

Sadie, An End of Life Story

At 20 years old still out and about and very loved, Sadie had hyperthyroidism. She would howl at night, confused, waking the household multiple times. Her guardians did not want to put her in isolation at the veterinary hospital to treat her thyroid with radiation, or put her on daily lifetime medication with its attendant side effects. Instead, they wanted to know what homeopathy could do. Treatment with her remedy helped Sadie relax, eased her confusion, and gave everyone a good night's sleep again. Her diarrhea also cleared up, which had plagued her for the past five months.

Sadie enjoyed another year of life without anything but the occasional homeopathic remedy, after which she died quietly in her favorite person's arms. Just before the end, Sadie reached out a paw to pull her guardian's hand close against her cheek.

One Cat's Whole Life with Homeopathy

Mame was suffering from chronic diarrhea at eight months old. A remedy stopped the diarrhea, and her guardian continued to use homeopathy over the following years. The same remedy, given infrequently, helped Mame with minor indispositions as she aged, such as eye discharge, bad breath, and vomiting. She is now doing well at 15 years old, and her last remedy dose was eight months ago.

Conclusion and Farewell

I hope that this book has piqued your interest in the wonderful healing modality of homeopathy. Our animals need us. Their vital forces are capable of healing, but they need medicine that engages that healing ability instead of suppressing symptoms. Once your eyes are open to the difference between suppression, palliation, and cure, I hope that you will begin to share your new knowledge with your family and your friends. The more we all learn the nature of true healing, the more we will change our hospitals and medical schools. Our physicians and veterinarians will begin to heal in the best sense of the word—working with the body's own knowledge of health and disease to transform our modern medical systems. And you are the beginning.

• • •

References Chapter 10

1. "Contents." *Vaccine Talk*. N.p., n.d. Web. 5 Sept. 2015. <http://vaccine.elehost.com/contents.htm>.
2. Fisher, S. G., L. Weber, and M. Carbone. "Cancer Risk Associated with Simian Virus 40 Contaminated Polio Vaccine." *PubMed.gov*. Cancer Cause and Prevention Program, n.d. Web. 5 Sept. 2015. <http://www.ncbi.nlm.nih.gov/pubmed/10472327>.

References

• • •

General Homeopathy Texts

Close S. *The Genius of Homoeopathy.* New Delhi, India: B. Jain Publishers; 1997.

Dooley TR. *Homeopathy: Beyond Flat Earth Medicine.* San Diego, CA: Timing Publication; 2002.

Dhawale LD. *Principles & Practice of Homoeopathy.* Bombay, India: S.Y. Chougule; 1994.

Farrington H. *Homoeopathy and Homoeopathic Prescribing.* New Delhi, India: B. Jain Publishers; 2001.

Gypser KH. *Kent's Minor Writings on Homoeopathy*. New Delhi, India: B. Jain Publishers; 1988.

Hahnemann S. *The Chronic Diseases: Their Peculiar Nature and Their Homoeopathic Cure.* Vol.1. Dresden and Leipzig, Germany: Arnold; 1828. [further reading on Hahnemann's theory of chronic diseases]

Hahnemann S. *Organon of Medicine, Sixth Edition*. Künzli J, Naudé A, and Pendleton P, eds. Blaine, WA: Cooper Publishing; 1982.

Hahnemann S. *Organon of the Medical Art, Sixth Edition*. O'Reilly WB, ed. Redmond, WA: Birdcage Books; 1996.

Henriques N. Crossroads to Cure: *The Homoeopath's Guide to Second Prescription*. St. Helena, CA: Totality Press; 1998.

Henriques N. *Release the Vital Force: The Exact Science and Art of*

Homeopathic Patient Examination. Napa Valley, CA: BookSurge; 2009.

Kent J. *Lectures on Homeopathic Philosophy*. Berkeley, CA: North Atlantic Books; 1979.

Roberts HA. *The Principles and Art of Cure by Homeopathy*. New Delhi, India: B. Jain Publishers; 1999.

Saxton, John and Peter Gregory. *Textbook of Veterinary Homeopathy*. Beaconsfield, UK: Beaconsfield Publishers, Ltd.; 2005.

Sherwood WW. *Kent's New Remedies, Clinical Cases, Lesser Writings, Aphorisms and Precepts.* New Delhi, India: B. Jain Publishers; 1921(reprint 1994).

Vithoulkas G. *The Science of Homeopathy*. New York, NY: Grove Press; 1980.

Yasgur J. *Yasgur's Homeopathic Dictionary.* Greenville, PA: Van Hoy Publishers; 1998.

• • •

Repertories

Boger CM. *Boenninghausen's Characteristics Materia Medica & Repertory.* Paharganj, New Delhi, India: B. Jain Publishers; 2003.

Kent JT. *Repertory of the Homoeopathic Materia Medica*. New Delhi, India: B. Jain Publishers; 1990.

Künzli J. *Kent's Repertorium Generale.* Berg am Starnberger, Germany: Barthel & Barthel Publishing; 1987.

Pitcairn R and Jensen W. *New World Veterinary Repertory.* Kandern,

Germany: Narayana Publishers; 2013.

Schroyens F. *Repertorium Homeopathicum Syntheticum* [edition 5.2]. New Delhi, India: B. Jain Publishers; 1993.

Zandvoort R. *Complete Repertory* from *MacRepertory.* [computer program] Version 4.5. San Rafael, CA: Kent Homeopathic Associates.

• • •

Materia Medicas

Allen TF. *The Encyclopedia of Pure Materia Medica: A Record of the Positive Effects of Drugs Upon the Healthy Human Organism*. New Delhi, India: B. Jain Publishers; 1982.

Boericke W. *Materia Medica with Repertory.* Santa Rosa, CA: Boericke & Tafel, Inc.; 1927.

Clarke JH. *Dictionary of Practical Materia Medica*. New Delhi, India: B. Jain Publishers; 1984.

Hahnemann S. *Materia Medica Pura.* New Delhi, India: B. Jain Publishers; 2002.

Hering C. *The Guiding Symptoms of Our Materia Medica*. Volumes [1-10]. Paharganj, New Delhi, India: B. Jain Publishers; 1995.

Kent J. *Lectures on Materia Medica*. New Delhi, India: B. Jain Publishers; 1993.

Lippe A. *Keynotes and Red Line Symptoms of the Materia Medica*. Paharganj, New Delhi, India: B. Jain Publishers; 1993.

Morrison R. *Desktop Guide to Keynotes and Confirmatory Symptoms.* Albany, CA: Hahnemann Clinic Publishing; 1993.

Vermeulen F. *Concordant Materia Medica.* Haarlem, The Netherlands: Emyrss Publishers; 1997.

Vermeulen F. *Synoptic Key* from *MacRepertory.* [computer program]. Version 3.9.7. San Rafael, CA: Kent Homeopathic Associates.

• • •

Guides to Natural Animal Care

Frazier A and Eckroate N. *The Natural Cat: The Comprehensive Guide to Optimum Care.* London, England: Penguin Books; 2008.

Hamilton D. *Homeopathic Care for Cats and Dogs: Small Doses for Small Animals.* Berkeley, CA: North Atlantic Books; 1999.

Pitcairn R and Pitcairn SH. Dr. Pitcairn's Complete Guide to Natural Health for Dogs & Cats. Emmaus, PA: Rodale Press, Inc.; 2005.

• • •

Homeopathy in First Aid

(as referred to in the chapter What Does Homeopathy Heal?)

Gilberd M. *Natural Remedies for Animal First Aid: With Full Animal herbal (Natural Remedies for Animals Series).* CreateSpace Independent Publishing Platform; 2013.

Walker K. *Homeopathic First Aid for Animals: Tales and Techniques from a Country Practitioner.* Rochester, VT: Healing Arts Press; 1998.

• • •

History of Homeopathy

Coulter HL. *Divided Legacy: The Conflict Between Homoeopathy and the American Medical Association*. Berkeley, CA: North Atlantic Books; 1982.

Winston J. *The Faces of Homœopathy an Illustrated History of the First 200 Years.* Tawa, Wellington, New Zealand: Great Auk Publishing; 1999.

• • •

Computer Programs

Synergy (software company, formerly Kent Homeopathic) http://www.kenthomeopathic.com/

Whole Health Now (homeopathic software, books, lectures) http://www.wholehealthnow.com/

• • •

Hand Repertorization Charts

http://homepage.isomedia.com/~homtut/Documents/RepSht1.pdf (condensed version)

http://homepage.isomedia.com/~homtut/Documents/RepSht2.pdf (expanded two page version)

Here's an example (incomplete) of a hand repertorization chart:

	Rubric 1	Rubric 2	Rubric 3	Rubric 4	Totals
acon.					
agar.					
alumn.					
anac.					
ant-c.					
ant-t.					
apis					
arg-n.....					

• • •

Vaccines

Coulter HL and Fisher B. *A Shot in the Dark: Why the P in the DPT Vaccination May Be Hazardous to Your Child's Health.* New York, NY: Penguin Group; 1991.

Miller NZ. *Vaccines: Are They Really Safe and Effective?* Santa Fe, NM: New Atlantean Press; 2008.

National Vaccine Information Center. http://www.nvic.org/

Neustaedter R. *The Immunization Decision: A Guide for Parents.* Berkeley, CA: North Atlantic Books; 1990.

• • •

Organizations

Academy of Veterinary Homeopathy (standards of homeopathic practice, referral listing of homeopathic veterinarians) http://theavh.org/

Animal Natural Health Center (referral listing of homeopathic veterinarians; advanced education for homeopathic veterinarians; books; lectures on tape) http://www.drpitcairn.com/

National Center for Homeopathy (publishes *Homeopathy Today*, which discusses legislative issues, clinical cases, and educational opportunities; also publishes a directory of homeopathic practitioners for humans and animals) http://www.nationalcenterforhomeopathy.org/

Pitcairn Institute of Veterinary Homeopathy (teaches the Professional Course in Veterinary Homeopathy for veterinarians) http://pivh.org/

• • •

Equine Natural Care

Dr. Joyce Harmany at http://harmanyequine.com/

• • •

Client Acceptance Form

(derived from the form provided by the Animal Natural Health Center)

I am honored that you are willing to trust me with the care of your animal. As you are likely already aware, my practice is not the usual. I offer consultation in the use of homeopathic remedies and nutrition (in the form of fresh food diets, vitamin and mineral supplementation, and food concentrates). I emphasize this form of treatment because I feel it is the most effective way of dealing with a wide variety of health problems that animals face. It is my opinion that homeopathic and nutritional therapy can be used to treat the same broad range of problems that are conventionally treated with drugs. It is also my experience that this is a very successful approach—one that I have studied and applied since 1994.

However, not every problem can be successfully resolved. Sometimes the disease is too advanced for my methods. Other times, I do not have the necessary knowledge or experience. Occasionally, my methods fail in spite of my best efforts. I say this not to discourage you, but rather to honestly communicate my skills and also my limitations.

It is important, as we start working together, that you realize, regardless of the nature of the problem your animal has and in spite of the diagnosis or prognosis that you have received from another practitioner, I am going to use the above-mentioned methods and no other in the treatment of your animal. If it becomes your decision to have conventional drug therapy or surgery, I will refer you to another practice that can provide this rather than do this myself. If it is my opinion that for the well-being of your animal you should receive care from another practitioner or by other methods, I will also refer you for this care rather than provide it myself.

If what has been presented here is acceptable to you and, indeed, what you wish for your animal, please sign the statement of acceptance that follows. Thank you!

Declaration of Acceptance:

I have read the above explanation of the type of treatment offered by [name of veterinarian]. I agree that this is what I want for my animal. I further state that I am not expecting any other treatment than what is described here.

Signed: [client's signature]

Index

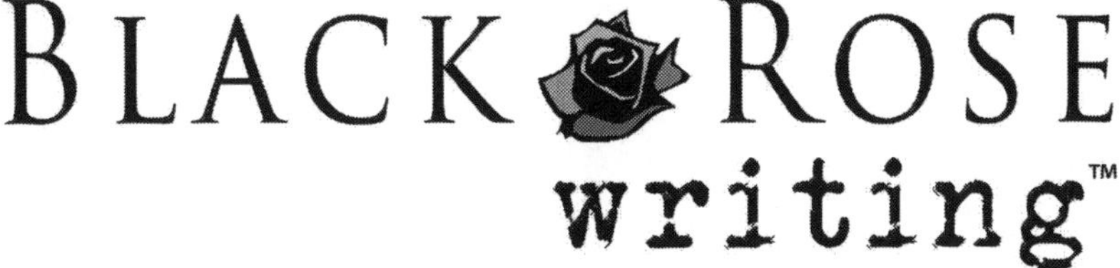
BLACK ROSE
writing™

Made in the USA
San Bernardino, CA
14 June 2018